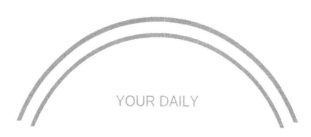

YOUR DAILY

FOOD & EXERCISE JOURNAL

START DATE:

_____

Exercise Activity: Hours || Minutes || Calories Burned

Measurements: Weight || Chest || Waist || Hips

How Do I Feel About
My Progress Today?

BREAKFAST			**LUNCH**		
TIME:			TIME:		
LOCATION:			LOCATION:		
FOOD ITEM	CALORIES	CARBS	FOOD ITEM	CALORIES	CARBS
TOTAL:			TOTAL:		
DINNER			**SNACK**		
TIME:			TIME:		
LOCATION:			LOCATION:		
FOOD ITEM	CALORIES	CARBS	FOOD ITEM	CALORIES	CARBS
TOTAL:			TOTAL:		

DATE _____

Exercise Activity: Hours ‖ Minutes ‖ Calories Burned

Measurements: Weight ‖ Chest ‖ Waist ‖ Hips

How Do I Feel About
My Progress Today?

BREAKFAST			LUNCH		
TIME:			TIME:		
LOCATION:			LOCATION:		
FOOD ITEM	CALORIES	CARBS	FOOD ITEM	CALORIES	CARBS
TOTAL:			TOTAL:		

DINNER			SNACK		
TIME:			TIME:		
LOCATION:			LOCATION:		
FOOD ITEM	CALORIES	CARBS	FOOD ITEM	CALORIES	CARBS
TOTAL:			TOTAL:		

DATE _____

Exercise Activity: Hours || Minutes || Calories Burned

_____

Measurements: Weight || Chest || Waist || Hips

_____

How Do I Feel About
My Progress Today?

BREAKFAST			LUNCH		
TIME:			TIME:		
LOCATION:			LOCATION:		
FOOD ITEM	CALORIES	CARBS	FOOD ITEM	CALORIES	CARBS
TOTAL:			TOTAL:		

DINNER			SNACK		
TIME:			TIME:		
LOCATION:			LOCATION:		
FOOD ITEM	CALORIES	CARBS	FOOD ITEM	CALORIES	CARBS
TOTAL:			TOTAL:		

DATE _____

Exercise Activity: Hours ‖ Minutes ‖ Calories Burned

Measurements: Weight ‖ Chest ‖ Waist ‖ Hips

How Do I Feel About
My Progress Today?

BREAKFAST			LUNCH		
TIME:			TIME:		
LOCATION:			LOCATION:		
FOOD ITEM	CALORIES	CARBS	FOOD ITEM	CALORIES	CARBS
TOTAL:			TOTAL:		

DINNER			SNACK		
TIME:			TIME:		
LOCATION:			LOCATION:		
FOOD ITEM	CALORIES	CARBS	FOOD ITEM	CALORIES	CARBS
TOTAL:			TOTAL:		

DATE _____

Exercise Activity: Hours || Minutes || Calories Burned

Measurements: Weight || Chest || Waist || Hips

How Do I Feel About
My Progress Today?

BREAKFAST			LUNCH		
TIME:			TIME:		
LOCATION:			LOCATION:		
FOOD ITEM	CALORIES	CARBS	FOOD ITEM	CALORIES	CARBS
TOTAL:			TOTAL:		

DINNER			SNACK		
TIME:			TIME:		
LOCATION:			LOCATION:		
FOOD ITEM	CALORIES	CARBS	FOOD ITEM	CALORIES	CARBS
TOTAL:			TOTAL:		

DATE _____

Exercise Activity: Hours || Minutes || Calories Burned

_____

Measurements: Weight || Chest || Waist || Hips

_____

How Do I Feel About
My Progress Today?

BREAKFAST			**LUNCH**		
TIME:			TIME:		
LOCATION:			LOCATION:		
FOOD ITEM	CALORIES	CARBS	FOOD ITEM	CALORIES	CARBS
TOTAL:			TOTAL:		

DINNER			**SNACK**		
TIME:			TIME:		
LOCATION:			LOCATION:		
FOOD ITEM	CALORIES	CARBS	FOOD ITEM	CALORIES	CARBS
TOTAL:			TOTAL:		

DATE _____

Exercise Activity: Hours ‖ Minutes ‖ Calories Burned

_____

Measurements: Weight ‖ Chest ‖ Waist ‖ Hips

_____

How Do I Feel About
My Progress Today?

BREAKFAST			LUNCH		
TIME:			TIME:		
LOCATION:			LOCATION:		
FOOD ITEM	CALORIES	CARBS	FOOD ITEM	CALORIES	CARBS
TOTAL:			TOTAL:		

DINNER			SNACK		
TIME:			TIME:		
LOCATION:			LOCATION:		
FOOD ITEM	CALORIES	CARBS	FOOD ITEM	CALORIES	CARBS
TOTAL:			TOTAL:		

Exercise Activity: Hours || Minutes || Calories Burned

Measurements: Weight || Chest || Waist || Hips

How Do I Feel About
My Progress Today?

BREAKFAST		
TIME:		
LOCATION:		
FOOD ITEM	CALORIES	CARBS
TOTAL:		

LUNCH		
TIME:		
LOCATION:		
FOOD ITEM	CALORIES	CARBS
TOTAL:		

DINNER		
TIME:		
LOCATION:		
FOOD ITEM	CALORIES	CARBS
TOTAL:		

SNACK		
TIME:		
LOCATION:		
FOOD ITEM	CALORIES	CARBS
TOTAL:		

DATE _____

Exercise Activity: Hours || Minutes || Calories Burned

Measurements: Weight || Chest || Waist || Hips

How Do I Feel About
My Progress Today?

BREAKFAST			LUNCH		
TIME:			TIME:		
LOCATION:			LOCATION:		
FOOD ITEM	CALORIES	CARBS	FOOD ITEM	CALORIES	CARBS
TOTAL:			TOTAL:		

DINNER			SNACK		
TIME:			TIME:		
LOCATION:			LOCATION:		
FOOD ITEM	CALORIES	CARBS	FOOD ITEM	CALORIES	CARBS
TOTAL:			TOTAL:		

DATE _____

Exercise Activity: Hours || Minutes || Calories Burned

Measurements: Weight || Chest || Waist || Hips

How Do I Feel About
My Progress Today?

BREAKFAST				LUNCH		
TIME:				TIME:		
LOCATION:				LOCATION:		
FOOD ITEM		CALORIES	CARBS	FOOD ITEM		CALORIES	CARBS
TOTAL:				TOTAL:		

DINNER				SNACK		
TIME:				TIME:		
LOCATION:				LOCATION:		
FOOD ITEM		CALORIES	CARBS	FOOD ITEM		CALORIES	CARBS
TOTAL:				TOTAL:		

Exercise Activity: Hours || Minutes || Calories Burned

_____

Measurements: Weight || Chest || Waist || Hips

_____

How Do I Feel About
My Progress Today?

BREAKFAST			LUNCH		
TIME:			TIME:		
LOCATION:			LOCATION:		
FOOD ITEM	CALORIES	CARBS	FOOD ITEM	CALORIES	CARBS
TOTAL:			TOTAL:		

DINNER			SNACK		
TIME:			TIME:		
LOCATION:			LOCATION:		
FOOD ITEM	CALORIES	CARBS	FOOD ITEM	CALORIES	CARBS
TOTAL:			TOTAL:		

DATE _____

Exercise Activity: Hours || Minutes || Calories Burned

Measurements: Weight || Chest || Waist || Hips

How Do I Feel About
My Progress Today?

BREAKFAST			LUNCH		
TIME:			TIME:		
LOCATION:			LOCATION:		
FOOD ITEM	CALORIES	CARBS	FOOD ITEM	CALORIES	CARBS
TOTAL:			TOTAL:		

DINNER			SNACK		
TIME:			TIME:		
LOCATION:			LOCATION:		
FOOD ITEM	CALORIES	CARBS	FOOD ITEM	CALORIES	CARBS
TOTAL:			TOTAL:		

Exercise Activity: Hours || Minutes || Calories Burned

_____

Measurements: Weight || Chest || Waist || Hips

_____

How Do I Feel About
My Progress Today?

BREAKFAST			LUNCH		
TIME:			TIME:		
LOCATION:			LOCATION:		
FOOD ITEM	CALORIES	CARBS	FOOD ITEM	CALORIES	CARBS
TOTAL:			TOTAL:		

DINNER			SNACK		
TIME:			TIME:		
LOCATION:			LOCATION:		
FOOD ITEM	CALORIES	CARBS	FOOD ITEM	CALORIES	CARBS
TOTAL:			TOTAL:		

DATE _____

Exercise Activity: Hours || Minutes || Calories Burned

Measurements: Weight || Chest || Waist || Hips

How Do I Feel About
My Progress Today?

BREAKFAST			LUNCH		
TIME:			TIME:		
LOCATION:			LOCATION:		
FOOD ITEM	CALORIES	CARBS	FOOD ITEM	CALORIES	CARBS
TOTAL:			TOTAL:		

DINNER			SNACK		
TIME:			TIME:		
LOCATION:			LOCATION:		
FOOD ITEM	CALORIES	CARBS	FOOD ITEM	CALORIES	CARBS
TOTAL:			TOTAL:		

| DATE | _____ |

Exercise Activity: Hours || Minutes || Calories Burned

Measurements: Weight || Chest || Waist || Hips

How Do I Feel About
My Progress Today?

BREAKFAST			LUNCH		
TIME:			TIME:		
LOCATION:			LOCATION:		
FOOD ITEM	CALORIES	CARBS	FOOD ITEM	CALORIES	CARBS
TOTAL:			TOTAL:		

DINNER			SNACK		
TIME:			TIME:		
LOCATION:			LOCATION:		
FOOD ITEM	CALORIES	CARBS	FOOD ITEM	CALORIES	CARBS
TOTAL:			TOTAL:		

Exercise Activity: Hours || Minutes || Calories Burned

Measurements: Weight || Chest || Waist || Hips

How Do I Feel About
My Progress Today?

BREAKFAST			LUNCH		
TIME:			TIME:		
LOCATION:			LOCATION:		
FOOD ITEM	CALORIES	CARBS	FOOD ITEM	CALORIES	CARBS
TOTAL:			TOTAL:		

DINNER			SNACK		
TIME:			TIME:		
LOCATION:			LOCATION:		
FOOD ITEM	CALORIES	CARBS	FOOD ITEM	CALORIES	CARBS
TOTAL:			TOTAL:		

DATE _____

Exercise Activity: Hours || Minutes || Calories Burned

Measurements: Weight || Chest || Waist || Hips

How Do I Feel About
My Progress Today?

BREAKFAST			LUNCH		
TIME:			TIME:		
LOCATION:			LOCATION:		
FOOD ITEM	CALORIES	CARBS	FOOD ITEM	CALORIES	CARBS
TOTAL:			TOTAL:		

DINNER			SNACK		
TIME:			TIME:		
LOCATION:			LOCATION:		
FOOD ITEM	CALORIES	CARBS	FOOD ITEM	CALORIES	CARBS
TOTAL:			TOTAL:		

DATE _____

Exercise Activity: Hours || Minutes || Calories Burned

Measurements: Weight || Chest || Waist || Hips

How Do I Feel About
My Progress Today?

BREAKFAST			LUNCH		
TIME:			TIME:		
LOCATION:			LOCATION:		
FOOD ITEM	CALORIES	CARBS	FOOD ITEM	CALORIES	CARBS
TOTAL:			TOTAL:		

DINNER			SNACK		
TIME:			TIME:		
LOCATION:			LOCATION:		
FOOD ITEM	CALORIES	CARBS	FOOD ITEM	CALORIES	CARBS
TOTAL:			TOTAL:		

DATE _____

Exercise Activity: Hours || Minutes || Calories Burned

_____

Measurements: Weight || Chest || Waist || Hips

_____

How Do I Feel About
My Progress Today?

BREAKFAST			LUNCH		
TIME:			TIME:		
LOCATION:			LOCATION:		
FOOD ITEM	CALORIES	CARBS	FOOD ITEM	CALORIES	CARBS
TOTAL:			TOTAL:		

DINNER			SNACK		
TIME:			TIME:		
LOCATION:			LOCATION:		
FOOD ITEM	CALORIES	CARBS	FOOD ITEM	CALORIES	CARBS
TOTAL:			TOTAL:		

DATE _____

Exercise Activity: Hours || Minutes || Calories Burned

Measurements: Weight || Chest || Waist || Hips

How Do I Feel About
My Progress Today?

BREAKFAST			LUNCH		
TIME:			TIME:		
LOCATION:			LOCATION:		
FOOD ITEM	CALORIES	CARBS	FOOD ITEM	CALORIES	CARBS
TOTAL:			TOTAL:		

DINNER			SNACK		
TIME:			TIME:		
LOCATION:			LOCATION:		
FOOD ITEM	CALORIES	CARBS	FOOD ITEM	CALORIES	CARBS
TOTAL:			TOTAL:		

DATE _____

Exercise Activity: Hours || Minutes || Calories Burned

Measurements: Weight || Chest || Waist || Hips

How Do I Feel About
My Progress Today?

BREAKFAST		
TIME:		
LOCATION:		
FOOD ITEM	CALORIES	CARBS
TOTAL:		

LUNCH		
TIME:		
LOCATION:		
FOOD ITEM	CALORIES	CARBS
TOTAL:		

DINNER		
TIME:		
LOCATION:		
FOOD ITEM	CALORIES	CARBS
TOTAL:		

SNACK		
TIME:		
LOCATION:		
FOOD ITEM	CALORIES	CARBS
TOTAL:		

Exercise Activity: Hours || Minutes || Calories Burned

Measurements: Weight || Chest || Waist || Hips

How Do I Feel About
My Progress Today?

BREAKFAST			LUNCH		
TIME:			TIME:		
LOCATION:			LOCATION:		
FOOD ITEM	CALORIES	CARBS	FOOD ITEM	CALORIES	CARBS
TOTAL:			TOTAL:		

DINNER			SNACK		
TIME:			TIME:		
LOCATION:			LOCATION:		
FOOD ITEM	CALORIES	CARBS	FOOD ITEM	CALORIES	CARBS
TOTAL:			TOTAL:		

DATE _____

Exercise Activity: Hours ‖ Minutes ‖ Calories Burned

Measurements: Weight ‖ Chest ‖ Waist ‖ Hips

How Do I Feel About
My Progress Today?

BREAKFAST			LUNCH		
TIME:			TIME:		
LOCATION:			LOCATION:		
FOOD ITEM	CALORIES	CARBS	FOOD ITEM	CALORIES	CARBS
TOTAL:			TOTAL:		

DINNER			SNACK		
TIME:			TIME:		
LOCATION:			LOCATION:		
FOOD ITEM	CALORIES	CARBS	FOOD ITEM	CALORIES	CARBS
TOTAL:			TOTAL:		

DATE _____

Exercise Activity: Hours ‖ Minutes ‖ Calories Burned

Measurements: Weight ‖ Chest ‖ Waist ‖ Hips

How Do I Feel About
My Progress Today?

BREAKFAST			LUNCH		
TIME:			TIME:		
LOCATION:			LOCATION:		
FOOD ITEM	CALORIES	CARBS	FOOD ITEM	CALORIES	CARBS
TOTAL:			TOTAL:		
DINNER			**SNACK**		
TIME:			TIME:		
LOCATION:			LOCATION:		
FOOD ITEM	CALORIES	CARBS	FOOD ITEM	CALORIES	CARBS
TOTAL:			TOTAL:		

DATE _____

Exercise Activity: Hours || Minutes || Calories Burned

Measurements: Weight || Chest || Waist || Hips

How Do I Feel About
My Progress Today?

BREAKFAST			LUNCH		
TIME:			TIME:		
LOCATION:			LOCATION:		
FOOD ITEM	CALORIES	CARBS	FOOD ITEM	CALORIES	CARBS
TOTAL:			TOTAL:		

DINNER			SNACK		
TIME:			TIME:		
LOCATION:			LOCATION:		
FOOD ITEM	CALORIES	CARBS	FOOD ITEM	CALORIES	CARBS
TOTAL:			TOTAL:		

DATE _____

Exercise Activity: Hours ‖ Minutes ‖ Calories Burned

_____

Measurements: Weight ‖ Chest ‖ Waist ‖ Hips

_____

How Do I Feel About
My Progress Today?

BREAKFAST			LUNCH		
TIME:			TIME:		
LOCATION:			LOCATION:		
FOOD ITEM	CALORIES	CARBS	FOOD ITEM	CALORIES	CARBS
TOTAL:			TOTAL:		

DINNER			SNACK		
TIME:			TIME:		
LOCATION:			LOCATION:		
FOOD ITEM	CALORIES	CARBS	FOOD ITEM	CALORIES	CARBS
TOTAL:			TOTAL:		

DATE _____

Exercise Activity: Hours || Minutes || Calories Burned

Measurements: Weight || Chest || Waist || Hips

How Do I Feel About My Progress Today?

BREAKFAST			LUNCH		
TIME:			TIME:		
LOCATION:			LOCATION:		
FOOD ITEM	CALORIES	CARBS	FOOD ITEM	CALORIES	CARBS
TOTAL:			TOTAL:		

DINNER			SNACK		
TIME:			TIME:		
LOCATION:			LOCATION:		
FOOD ITEM	CALORIES	CARBS	FOOD ITEM	CALORIES	CARBS
TOTAL:			TOTAL:		

DATE _____

Exercise Activity: Hours || Minutes || Calories Burned

Measurements: Weight || Chest || Waist || Hips

How Do I Feel About
My Progress Today?

BREAKFAST			LUNCH		
TIME:			TIME:		
LOCATION:			LOCATION:		
FOOD ITEM	CALORIES	CARBS	FOOD ITEM	CALORIES	CARBS
TOTAL:			TOTAL:		

DINNER			SNACK		
TIME:			TIME:		
LOCATION:			LOCATION:		
FOOD ITEM	CALORIES	CARBS	FOOD ITEM	CALORIES	CARBS
TOTAL:			TOTAL:		

Exercise Activity: Hours || Minutes || Calories Burned

Measurements: Weight || Chest || Waist || Hips

How Do I Feel About
My Progress Today?

BREAKFAST			LUNCH		
TIME:			TIME:		
LOCATION:			LOCATION:		
FOOD ITEM	CALORIES	CARBS	FOOD ITEM	CALORIES	CARBS
TOTAL:			TOTAL:		

DINNER			SNACK		
TIME:			TIME:		
LOCATION:			LOCATION:		
FOOD ITEM	CALORIES	CARBS	FOOD ITEM	CALORIES	CARBS
TOTAL:			TOTAL:		

Exercise Activity: Hours ‖ Minutes ‖ Calories Burned

Measurements: Weight ‖ Chest ‖ Waist ‖ Hips

How Do I Feel About
My Progress Today?

BREAKFAST			
TIME:			
LOCATION:			
FOOD ITEM		CALORIES	CARBS
TOTAL:			

LUNCH			
TIME:			
LOCATION:			
FOOD ITEM		CALORIES	CARBS
TOTAL:			

DINNER			
TIME:			
LOCATION:			
FOOD ITEM		CALORIES	CARBS
TOTAL:			

SNACK			
TIME:			
LOCATION:			
FOOD ITEM		CALORIES	CARBS
TOTAL:			

DATE _____

Exercise Activity: Hours || Minutes || Calories Burned

Measurements: Weight || Chest || Waist || Hips

How Do I Feel About
My Progress Today?

BREAKFAST			LUNCH		
TIME:			TIME:		
LOCATION:			LOCATION:		
FOOD ITEM	CALORIES	CARBS	FOOD ITEM	CALORIES	CARBS
TOTAL:			TOTAL:		

DINNER			SNACK		
TIME:			TIME:		
LOCATION:			LOCATION:		
FOOD ITEM	CALORIES	CARBS	FOOD ITEM	CALORIES	CARBS
TOTAL:			TOTAL:		

DATE _____

Exercise Activity: Hours || Minutes || Calories Burned

Measurements: Weight || Chest || Waist || Hips

How Do I Feel About
My Progress Today?

BREAKFAST			LUNCH		
TIME:			TIME:		
LOCATION:			LOCATION:		
FOOD ITEM	CALORIES	CARBS	FOOD ITEM	CALORIES	CARBS
TOTAL:			TOTAL:		

DINNER			SNACK		
TIME:			TIME:		
LOCATION:			LOCATION:		
FOOD ITEM	CALORIES	CARBS	FOOD ITEM	CALORIES	CARBS
TOTAL:			TOTAL:		

DATE _____

Exercise Activity: Hours || Minutes || Calories Burned

Measurements: Weight || Chest || Waist || Hips

How Do I Feel About
My Progress Today?

BREAKFAST			LUNCH		
TIME:			TIME:		
LOCATION:			LOCATION:		
FOOD ITEM	CALORIES	CARBS	FOOD ITEM	CALORIES	CARBS
TOTAL:			TOTAL:		

DINNER			SNACK		
TIME:			TIME:		
LOCATION:			LOCATION:		
FOOD ITEM	CALORIES	CARBS	FOOD ITEM	CALORIES	CARBS
TOTAL:			TOTAL:		

Exercise Activity: Hours || Minutes || Calories Burned

Measurements: Weight || Chest || Waist || Hips

How Do I Feel About
My Progress Today?

BREAKFAST			LUNCH		
TIME:			TIME:		
LOCATION:			LOCATION:		
FOOD ITEM	CALORIES	CARBS	FOOD ITEM	CALORIES	CARBS
TOTAL:			TOTAL:		

DINNER			SNACK		
TIME:			TIME:		
LOCATION:			LOCATION:		
FOOD ITEM	CALORIES	CARBS	FOOD ITEM	CALORIES	CARBS
TOTAL:			TOTAL:		

Exercise Activity: Hours || Minutes || Calories Burned

Measurements: Weight || Chest || Waist || Hips

How Do I Feel About
My Progress Today?

BREAKFAST			LUNCH		
TIME:			TIME:		
LOCATION:			LOCATION:		
FOOD ITEM	CALORIES	CARBS	FOOD ITEM	CALORIES	CARBS
TOTAL:			TOTAL:		

DINNER			SNACK		
TIME:			TIME:		
LOCATION:			LOCATION:		
FOOD ITEM	CALORIES	CARBS	FOOD ITEM	CALORIES	CARBS
TOTAL:			TOTAL:		

DATE _____

Exercise Activity: Hours || Minutes || Calories Burned

Measurements: Weight || Chest || Waist || Hips

How Do I Feel About
My Progress Today?

BREAKFAST			LUNCH		
TIME:			TIME:		
LOCATION:			LOCATION:		
FOOD ITEM	CALORIES	CARBS	FOOD ITEM	CALORIES	CARBS
TOTAL:			TOTAL:		

DINNER			SNACK		
TIME:			TIME:		
LOCATION:			LOCATION:		
FOOD ITEM	CALORIES	CARBS	FOOD ITEM	CALORIES	CARBS
TOTAL:			TOTAL:		

DATE _____

Exercise Activity:　Hours　‖　Minutes　‖　Calories Burned

Measurements: Weight　‖　Chest　‖　Waist　‖　Hips

How Do I Feel About My Progress Today?

BREAKFAST			LUNCH		
TIME:			TIME:		
LOCATION:			LOCATION:		
FOOD ITEM	| CALORIES	| CARBS	FOOD ITEM	| CALORIES	| CARBS
TOTAL:			TOTAL:		

DINNER			SNACK		
TIME:			TIME:		
LOCATION:			LOCATION:		
FOOD ITEM	| CALORIES	| CARBS	FOOD ITEM	| CALORIES	| CARBS
TOTAL:			TOTAL:		

DATE _____

Exercise Activity: Hours || Minutes || Calories Burned

Measurements: Weight || Chest || Waist || Hips

How Do I Feel About
My Progress Today?

BREAKFAST			LUNCH		
TIME:			TIME:		
LOCATION:			LOCATION:		
FOOD ITEM	CALORIES	CARBS	FOOD ITEM	CALORIES	CARBS
TOTAL:			TOTAL:		

DINNER			SNACK		
TIME:			TIME:		
LOCATION:			LOCATION:		
FOOD ITEM	CALORIES	CARBS	FOOD ITEM	CALORIES	CARBS
TOTAL:			TOTAL:		

DATE _____

Exercise Activity: Hours || Minutes || Calories Burned

Measurements: Weight || Chest || Waist || Hips

How Do I Feel About
My Progress Today?

BREAKFAST				LUNCH		
TIME:				TIME:		
LOCATION:				LOCATION:		
FOOD ITEM		CALORIES	CARBS	FOOD ITEM		CALORIES	CARBS
TOTAL:				TOTAL:		

DINNER				SNACK		
TIME:				TIME:		
LOCATION:				LOCATION:		
FOOD ITEM		CALORIES	CARBS	FOOD ITEM		CALORIES	CARBS
TOTAL:				TOTAL:		

DATE _____

Exercise Activity: Hours || Minutes || Calories Burned

Measurements: Weight || Chest || Waist || Hips

How Do I Feel About
My Progress Today?

BREAKFAST			LUNCH		
TIME:			TIME:		
LOCATION:			LOCATION:		
FOOD ITEM	CALORIES	CARBS	FOOD ITEM	CALORIES	CARBS
TOTAL:			TOTAL:		

DINNER			SNACK		
TIME:			TIME:		
LOCATION:			LOCATION:		
FOOD ITEM	CALORIES	CARBS	FOOD ITEM	CALORIES	CARBS
TOTAL:			TOTAL:		

Exercise Activity: Hours || Minutes || Calories Burned

Measurements: Weight || Chest || Waist || Hips

How Do I Feel About
My Progress Today?

BREAKFAST			LUNCH		
TIME:			TIME:		
LOCATION:			LOCATION:		
FOOD ITEM	CALORIES	CARBS	FOOD ITEM	CALORIES	CARBS
TOTAL:			TOTAL:		

DINNER			SNACK		
TIME:			TIME:		
LOCATION:			LOCATION:		
FOOD ITEM	CALORIES	CARBS	FOOD ITEM	CALORIES	CARBS
TOTAL:			TOTAL:		

DATE _____

Exercise Activity: Hours ‖ Minutes ‖ Calories Burned

Measurements: Weight ‖ Chest ‖ Waist ‖ Hips

How Do I Feel About
My Progress Today?

BREAKFAST		
TIME:		
LOCATION:		
FOOD ITEM	CALORIES	CARBS
TOTAL:		

LUNCH		
TIME:		
LOCATION:		
FOOD ITEM	CALORIES	CARBS
TOTAL:		

DINNER		
TIME:		
LOCATION:		
FOOD ITEM	CALORIES	CARBS
TOTAL:		

SNACK		
TIME:		
LOCATION:		
FOOD ITEM	CALORIES	CARBS
TOTAL:		

Exercise Activity: Hours || Minutes || Calories Burned

Measurements: Weight || Chest || Waist || Hips

How Do I Feel About My Progress Today?

BREAKFAST			LUNCH		
TIME:			TIME:		
LOCATION:			LOCATION:		
FOOD ITEM	CALORIES	CARBS	FOOD ITEM	CALORIES	CARBS
TOTAL:			TOTAL:		

DINNER			SNACK		
TIME:			TIME:		
LOCATION:			LOCATION:		
FOOD ITEM	CALORIES	CARBS	FOOD ITEM	CALORIES	CARBS
TOTAL:			TOTAL:		

DATE _____

Exercise Activity: Hours || Minutes || Calories Burned

Measurements: Weight || Chest || Waist || Hips

How Do I Feel About
My Progress Today?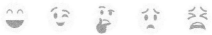

BREAKFAST	CALORIES	CARBS	LUNCH	CALORIES	CARBS
TIME:			TIME:		
LOCATION:			LOCATION:		
FOOD ITEM	CALORIES	CARBS	FOOD ITEM	CALORIES	CARBS
TOTAL:			TOTAL:		

DINNER	CALORIES	CARBS	SNACK	CALORIES	CARBS
TIME:			TIME:		
LOCATION:			LOCATION:		
FOOD ITEM	CALORIES	CARBS	FOOD ITEM	CALORIES	CARBS
TOTAL:			TOTAL:		

DATE _____

Exercise Activity:　Hours　‖　Minutes　‖　Calories Burned

Measurements: Weight　‖　Chest　‖　Waist　‖　Hips

How Do I Feel About
My Progress Today?

BREAKFAST			LUNCH		
TIME:			TIME:		
LOCATION:			LOCATION:		
FOOD ITEM	CALORIES	CARBS	FOOD ITEM	CALORIES	CARBS
TOTAL:			TOTAL:		

DINNER			SNACK		
TIME:			TIME:		
LOCATION:			LOCATION:		
FOOD ITEM	CALORIES	CARBS	FOOD ITEM	CALORIES	CARBS
TOTAL:			TOTAL:		

DATE _____

Exercise Activity: Hours || Minutes || Calories Burned

Measurements: Weight || Chest || Waist || Hips

How Do I Feel About My Progress Today?

BREAKFAST			LUNCH		
TIME:			TIME:		
LOCATION:			LOCATION:		
FOOD ITEM	CALORIES	CARBS	FOOD ITEM	CALORIES	CARBS
TOTAL:			TOTAL:		

DINNER			SNACK		
TIME:			TIME:		
LOCATION:			LOCATION:		
FOOD ITEM	CALORIES	CARBS	FOOD ITEM	CALORIES	CARBS
TOTAL:			TOTAL:		

DATE _____

Exercise Activity: Hours || Minutes || Calories Burned

Measurements: Weight || Chest || Waist || Hips

How Do I Feel About My Progress Today?

BREAKFAST			LUNCH		
TIME:			TIME:		
LOCATION:			LOCATION:		
FOOD ITEM	CALORIES	CARBS	FOOD ITEM	CALORIES	CARBS
TOTAL:			TOTAL:		

DINNER			SNACK		
TIME:			TIME:		
LOCATION:			LOCATION:		
FOOD ITEM	CALORIES	CARBS	FOOD ITEM	CALORIES	CARBS
TOTAL:			TOTAL:		

Exercise Activity: Hours ‖ Minutes ‖ Calories Burned

Measurements: Weight ‖ Chest ‖ Waist ‖ Hips

How Do I Feel About
My Progress Today?

BREAKFAST			LUNCH		
TIME:			TIME:		
LOCATION:			LOCATION:		
FOOD ITEM	CALORIES	CARBS	FOOD ITEM	CALORIES	CARBS
TOTAL:			TOTAL:		

DINNER			SNACK		
TIME:			TIME:		
LOCATION:			LOCATION:		
FOOD ITEM	CALORIES	CARBS	FOOD ITEM	CALORIES	CARBS
TOTAL:			TOTAL:		

DATE _____

Exercise Activity: Hours ‖ Minutes ‖ Calories Burned

Measurements: Weight ‖ Chest ‖ Waist ‖ Hips

How Do I Feel About My Progress Today?

BREAKFAST			LUNCH		
TIME:			TIME:		
LOCATION:			LOCATION:		
FOOD ITEM	CALORIES	CARBS	FOOD ITEM	CALORIES	CARBS
TOTAL:			TOTAL:		

DINNER			SNACK		
TIME:			TIME:		
LOCATION:			LOCATION:		
FOOD ITEM	CALORIES	CARBS	FOOD ITEM	CALORIES	CARBS
TOTAL:			TOTAL:		

DATE _____

Exercise Activity: Hours || Minutes || Calories Burned

_____

Measurements: Weight || Chest || Waist || Hips

_____

How Do I Feel About
My Progress Today?

BREAKFAST			LUNCH		
TIME:			TIME:		
LOCATION:			LOCATION:		
FOOD ITEM	CALORIES	CARBS	FOOD ITEM	CALORIES	CARBS
TOTAL:			TOTAL:		

DINNER			SNACK		
TIME:			TIME:		
LOCATION:			LOCATION:		
FOOD ITEM	CALORIES	CARBS	FOOD ITEM	CALORIES	CARBS
TOTAL:			TOTAL:		

DATE _____

Exercise Activity: Hours || Minutes || Calories Burned

Measurements: Weight || Chest || Waist || Hips

How Do I Feel About
My Progress Today?

BREAKFAST			**LUNCH**		
TIME:			TIME:		
LOCATION:			LOCATION:		
FOOD ITEM	CALORIES	CARBS	FOOD ITEM	CALORIES	CARBS
TOTAL:			TOTAL:		
DINNER			**SNACK**		
TIME:			TIME:		
LOCATION:			LOCATION:		
FOOD ITEM	CALORIES	CARBS	FOOD ITEM	CALORIES	CARBS
TOTAL:			TOTAL:		

DATE _____

Exercise Activity: Hours || Minutes || Calories Burned

Measurements: Weight || Chest || Waist || Hips

How Do I Feel About
My Progress Today?

BREAKFAST			LUNCH		
TIME:			TIME:		
LOCATION:			LOCATION:		
FOOD ITEM	CALORIES	CARBS	FOOD ITEM	CALORIES	CARBS
TOTAL:			TOTAL:		

DINNER			SNACK		
TIME:			TIME:		
LOCATION:			LOCATION:		
FOOD ITEM	CALORIES	CARBS	FOOD ITEM	CALORIES	CARBS
TOTAL:			TOTAL:		

Exercise Activity: Hours || Minutes || Calories Burned

Measurements: Weight || Chest || Waist || Hips

How Do I Feel About
My Progress Today?

BREAKFAST			LUNCH		
TIME:			TIME:		
LOCATION:			LOCATION:		
FOOD ITEM	CALORIES	CARBS	FOOD ITEM	CALORIES	CARBS
TOTAL:			TOTAL:		

DINNER			SNACK		
TIME:			TIME:		
LOCATION:			LOCATION:		
FOOD ITEM	CALORIES	CARBS	FOOD ITEM	CALORIES	CARBS
TOTAL:			TOTAL:		

DATE _____

Exercise Activity: Hours || Minutes || Calories Burned

Measurements: Weight || Chest || Waist || Hips

How Do I Feel About
My Progress Today?

BREAKFAST				LUNCH		
TIME:				TIME:		
LOCATION:				LOCATION:		
FOOD ITEM	| CALORIES	| CARBS		FOOD ITEM	| CALORIES	| CARBS
TOTAL:				TOTAL:		

DINNER				SNACK		
TIME:				TIME:		
LOCATION:				LOCATION:		
FOOD ITEM	| CALORIES	| CARBS		FOOD ITEM	| CALORIES	| CARBS
TOTAL:				TOTAL:		

Exercise Activity: Hours || Minutes || Calories Burned

Measurements: Weight || Chest || Waist || Hips

How Do I Feel About
My Progress Today?

BREAKFAST

TIME:

LOCATION:

FOOD ITEM		CALORIES	CARBS
TOTAL:			

LUNCH

TIME:

LOCATION:

FOOD ITEM		CALORIES	CARBS
TOTAL:			

DINNER

TIME:

LOCATION:

FOOD ITEM		CALORIES	CARBS
TOTAL:			

SNACK

TIME:

LOCATION:

FOOD ITEM		CALORIES	CARBS
TOTAL:			

DATE _____

Exercise Activity: Hours ‖ Minutes ‖ Calories Burned

Measurements: Weight ‖ Chest ‖ Waist ‖ Hips

How Do I Feel About
My Progress Today?

BREAKFAST			LUNCH		
TIME:			TIME:		
LOCATION:			LOCATION:		
FOOD ITEM	CALORIES	CARBS	FOOD ITEM	CALORIES	CARBS
TOTAL:			TOTAL:		

DINNER			SNACK		
TIME:			TIME:		
LOCATION:			LOCATION:		
FOOD ITEM	CALORIES	CARBS	FOOD ITEM	CALORIES	CARBS
TOTAL:			TOTAL:		

Exercise Activity: Hours || Minutes || Calories Burned

Measurements: Weight || Chest || Waist || Hips

How Do I Feel About My Progress Today?

BREAKFAST			**LUNCH**		
TIME:			TIME:		
LOCATION:			LOCATION:		
FOOD ITEM	CALORIES	CARBS	FOOD ITEM	CALORIES	CARBS
TOTAL:			TOTAL:		
DINNER			**SNACK**		
TIME:			TIME:		
LOCATION:			LOCATION:		
FOOD ITEM	CALORIES	CARBS	FOOD ITEM	CALORIES	CARBS
TOTAL:			TOTAL:		

DATE _____

Exercise Activity: Hours || Minutes || Calories Burned

Measurements: Weight || Chest || Waist || Hips

How Do I Feel About
My Progress Today?

BREAKFAST			LUNCH		
TIME:			TIME:		
LOCATION:			LOCATION:		
FOOD ITEM	CALORIES	CARBS	FOOD ITEM	CALORIES	CARBS
TOTAL:			TOTAL:		

DINNER			SNACK		
TIME:			TIME:		
LOCATION:			LOCATION:		
FOOD ITEM	CALORIES	CARBS	FOOD ITEM	CALORIES	CARBS
TOTAL:			TOTAL:		

DATE _____

Exercise Activity: Hours ‖ Minutes ‖ Calories Burned

Measurements: Weight ‖ Chest ‖ Waist ‖ Hips

How Do I Feel About My Progress Today?

BREAKFAST			LUNCH		
TIME:			TIME:		
LOCATION:			LOCATION:		
FOOD ITEM	CALORIES	CARBS	FOOD ITEM	CALORIES	CARBS
TOTAL:			TOTAL:		

DINNER			SNACK		
TIME:			TIME:		
LOCATION:			LOCATION:		
FOOD ITEM	CALORIES	CARBS	FOOD ITEM	CALORIES	CARBS
TOTAL:			TOTAL:		

DATE _____

Exercise Activity: Hours ‖ Minutes ‖ Calories Burned

Measurements: Weight ‖ Chest ‖ Waist ‖ Hips

How Do I Feel About My Progress Today?

BREAKFAST				LUNCH			
TIME:				TIME:			
LOCATION:				LOCATION:			
FOOD ITEM		CALORIES	CARBS	FOOD ITEM		CALORIES	CARBS
TOTAL:				TOTAL:			

DINNER				SNACK			
TIME:				TIME:			
LOCATION:				LOCATION:			
FOOD ITEM		CALORIES	CARBS	FOOD ITEM		CALORIES	CARBS
TOTAL:				TOTAL:			

Exercise Activity: Hours || Minutes || Calories Burned

Measurements: Weight || Chest || Waist || Hips

How Do I Feel About
My Progress Today?

BREAKFAST			LUNCH		
TIME:			TIME:		
LOCATION:			LOCATION:		
FOOD ITEM	CALORIES	CARBS	FOOD ITEM	CALORIES	CARBS
TOTAL:			TOTAL:		

DINNER			SNACK		
TIME:			TIME:		
LOCATION:			LOCATION:		
FOOD ITEM	CALORIES	CARBS	FOOD ITEM	CALORIES	CARBS
TOTAL:			TOTAL:		

Exercise Activity: Hours || Minutes || Calories Burned

Measurements: Weight || Chest || Waist || Hips

How Do I Feel About
My Progress Today?

BREAKFAST			LUNCH		
TIME:			TIME:		
LOCATION:			LOCATION:		
FOOD ITEM	CALORIES	CARBS	FOOD ITEM	CALORIES	CARBS
TOTAL:			TOTAL:		

DINNER			SNACK		
TIME:			TIME:		
LOCATION:			LOCATION:		
FOOD ITEM	CALORIES	CARBS	FOOD ITEM	CALORIES	CARBS
TOTAL:			TOTAL:		

Exercise Activity: Hours || Minutes || Calories Burned

Measurements: Weight || Chest || Waist || Hips

How Do I Feel About
My Progress Today?

BREAKFAST			LUNCH		
TIME:			TIME:		
LOCATION:			LOCATION:		
FOOD ITEM	CALORIES	CARBS	FOOD ITEM	CALORIES	CARBS
TOTAL:			TOTAL:		

DINNER			SNACK		
TIME:			TIME:		
LOCATION:			LOCATION:		
FOOD ITEM	CALORIES	CARBS	FOOD ITEM	CALORIES	CARBS
TOTAL:			TOTAL:		

Exercise Activity: Hours || Minutes || Calories Burned

Measurements: Weight || Chest || Waist || Hips

How Do I Feel About
My Progress Today?

BREAKFAST		
TIME:		
LOCATION:		
FOOD ITEM	CALORIES	CARBS
TOTAL:		

LUNCH		
TIME:		
LOCATION:		
FOOD ITEM	CALORIES	CARBS
TOTAL:		

DINNER		
TIME:		
LOCATION:		
FOOD ITEM	CALORIES	CARBS
TOTAL:		

SNACK		
TIME:		
LOCATION:		
FOOD ITEM	CALORIES	CARBS
TOTAL:		

DATE _____

Exercise Activity: Hours || Minutes || Calories Burned

Measurements: Weight || Chest || Waist || Hips

How Do I Feel About
My Progress Today?

BREAKFAST			LUNCH		
TIME:			TIME:		
LOCATION:			LOCATION:		
FOOD ITEM	CALORIES	CARBS	FOOD ITEM	CALORIES	CARBS
TOTAL:			TOTAL:		

DINNER			SNACK		
TIME:			TIME:		
LOCATION:			LOCATION:		
FOOD ITEM	CALORIES	CARBS	FOOD ITEM	CALORIES	CARBS
TOTAL:			TOTAL:		

DATE _____

Exercise Activity: Hours || Minutes || Calories Burned

Measurements: Weight || Chest || Waist || Hips

How Do I Feel About My Progress Today?

BREAKFAST				LUNCH			
TIME:				TIME:			
LOCATION:				LOCATION:			
FOOD ITEM		CALORIES	CARBS	FOOD ITEM		CALORIES	CARBS
TOTAL:				TOTAL:			

DINNER				SNACK			
TIME:				TIME:			
LOCATION:				LOCATION:			
FOOD ITEM		CALORIES	CARBS	FOOD ITEM		CALORIES	CARBS
TOTAL:				TOTAL:			

DATE _____

Exercise Activity: Hours || Minutes || Calories Burned

Measurements: Weight || Chest || Waist || Hips

How Do I Feel About
My Progress Today?

BREAKFAST			LUNCH		
TIME:			TIME:		
LOCATION:			LOCATION:		
FOOD ITEM	CALORIES	CARBS	FOOD ITEM	CALORIES	CARBS
TOTAL:			TOTAL:		

DINNER			SNACK		
TIME:			TIME:		
LOCATION:			LOCATION:		
FOOD ITEM	CALORIES	CARBS	FOOD ITEM	CALORIES	CARBS
TOTAL:			TOTAL:		

DATE _____

Exercise Activity: Hours ‖ Minutes ‖ Calories Burned

Measurements: Weight ‖ Chest ‖ Waist ‖ Hips

How Do I Feel About My Progress Today?

BREAKFAST			LUNCH		
TIME:			TIME:		
LOCATION:			LOCATION:		
FOOD ITEM	CALORIES	CARBS	FOOD ITEM	CALORIES	CARBS
TOTAL:			TOTAL:		

DINNER			SNACK		
TIME:			TIME:		
LOCATION:			LOCATION:		
FOOD ITEM	CALORIES	CARBS	FOOD ITEM	CALORIES	CARBS
TOTAL:			TOTAL:		

DATE _____

Exercise Activity: Hours || Minutes || Calories Burned

Measurements: Weight || Chest || Waist || Hips

How Do I Feel About
My Progress Today?

BREAKFAST			LUNCH		
TIME:			TIME:		
LOCATION:			LOCATION:		
FOOD ITEM	CALORIES	CARBS	FOOD ITEM	CALORIES	CARBS
TOTAL:			TOTAL:		

DINNER			SNACK		
TIME:			TIME:		
LOCATION:			LOCATION:		
FOOD ITEM	CALORIES	CARBS	FOOD ITEM	CALORIES	CARBS
TOTAL:			TOTAL:		

Exercise Activity: Hours || Minutes || Calories Burned

Measurements: Weight || Chest || Waist || Hips

How Do I Feel About
My Progress Today?

BREAKFAST		
TIME:		
LOCATION:		
FOOD ITEM	CALORIES	CARBS
TOTAL:		

LUNCH		
TIME:		
LOCATION:		
FOOD ITEM	CALORIES	CARBS
TOTAL:		

DINNER		
TIME:		
LOCATION:		
FOOD ITEM	CALORIES	CARBS
TOTAL:		

SNACK		
TIME:		
LOCATION:		
FOOD ITEM	CALORIES	CARBS
TOTAL:		

Exercise Activity: Hours || Minutes || Calories Burned

_____

Measurements: Weight || Chest || Waist || Hips

_____

How Do I Feel About
My Progress Today?

BREAKFAST			LUNCH		
TIME:			TIME:		
LOCATION:			LOCATION:		
FOOD ITEM	CALORIES	CARBS	FOOD ITEM	CALORIES	CARBS
TOTAL:			TOTAL:		
DINNER			**SNACK**		
TIME:			TIME:		
LOCATION:			LOCATION:		
FOOD ITEM	CALORIES	CARBS	FOOD ITEM	CALORIES	CARBS
TOTAL:			TOTAL:		

Exercise Activity: Hours || Minutes || Calories Burned

Measurements: Weight || Chest || Waist || Hips

How Do I Feel About
My Progress Today?

BREAKFAST			**LUNCH**		
TIME:			TIME:		
LOCATION:			LOCATION:		
FOOD ITEM	CALORIES	CARBS	FOOD ITEM	CALORIES	CARBS
TOTAL:			TOTAL:		
DINNER			**SNACK**		
TIME:			TIME:		
LOCATION:			LOCATION:		
FOOD ITEM	CALORIES	CARBS	FOOD ITEM	CALORIES	CARBS
TOTAL:			TOTAL:		

DATE _____

Exercise Activity: Hours || Minutes || Calories Burned

Measurements: Weight || Chest || Waist || Hips

How Do I Feel About
My Progress Today?

BREAKFAST			LUNCH		
TIME:			TIME:		
LOCATION:			LOCATION:		
FOOD ITEM	CALORIES	CARBS	FOOD ITEM	CALORIES	CARBS
TOTAL:			TOTAL:		

DINNER			SNACK		
TIME:			TIME:		
LOCATION:			LOCATION:		
FOOD ITEM	CALORIES	CARBS	FOOD ITEM	CALORIES	CARBS
TOTAL:			TOTAL:		

DATE _____

Exercise Activity: Hours || Minutes || Calories Burned

Measurements: Weight || Chest || Waist || Hips

How Do I Feel About My Progress Today?

BREAKFAST			LUNCH		
TIME:			TIME:		
LOCATION:			LOCATION:		
FOOD ITEM	CALORIES	CARBS	FOOD ITEM	CALORIES	CARBS
TOTAL:			TOTAL:		

DINNER			SNACK		
TIME:			TIME:		
LOCATION:			LOCATION:		
FOOD ITEM	CALORIES	CARBS	FOOD ITEM	CALORIES	CARBS
TOTAL:			TOTAL:		

Exercise Activity: Hours || Minutes || Calories Burned

Measurements: Weight || Chest || Waist || Hips

How Do I Feel About
My Progress Today?

BREAKFAST				LUNCH		
TIME:				TIME:		
LOCATION:				LOCATION:		
FOOD ITEM		CALORIES	CARBS	FOOD ITEM		CALORIES	CARBS
TOTAL:				TOTAL:		

DINNER				SNACK		
TIME:				TIME:		
LOCATION:				LOCATION:		
FOOD ITEM		CALORIES	CARBS	FOOD ITEM		CALORIES	CARBS
TOTAL:				TOTAL:		

DATE _____

Exercise Activity: Hours || Minutes || Calories Burned

Measurements: Weight || Chest || Waist || Hips

How Do I Feel About
My Progress Today?

BREAKFAST				LUNCH		
TIME:				TIME:		
LOCATION:				LOCATION:		
FOOD ITEM		CALORIES	CARBS	FOOD ITEM		CALORIES	CARBS
TOTAL:				TOTAL:		

DINNER				SNACK		
TIME:				TIME:		
LOCATION:				LOCATION:		
FOOD ITEM		CALORIES	CARBS	FOOD ITEM		CALORIES	CARBS
TOTAL:				TOTAL:		

Exercise Activity: Hours ‖ Minutes ‖ Calories Burned

Measurements: Weight ‖ Chest ‖ Waist ‖ Hips

How Do I Feel About My Progress Today?

BREAKFAST			**LUNCH**		
TIME:			TIME:		
LOCATION:			LOCATION:		
FOOD ITEM	CALORIES	CARBS	FOOD ITEM	CALORIES	CARBS
TOTAL:			TOTAL:		

DINNER			**SNACK**		
TIME:			TIME:		
LOCATION:			LOCATION:		
FOOD ITEM	CALORIES	CARBS	FOOD ITEM	CALORIES	CARBS
TOTAL:			TOTAL:		

Exercise Activity: Hours || Minutes || Calories Burned

Measurements: Weight || Chest || Waist || Hips

How Do I Feel About
My Progress Today?

BREAKFAST				**LUNCH**		
TIME:				TIME:		
LOCATION:				LOCATION:		
FOOD ITEM	CALORIES	CARBS		FOOD ITEM	CALORIES	CARBS
TOTAL:				TOTAL:		

DINNER				**SNACK**		
TIME:				TIME:		
LOCATION:				LOCATION:		
FOOD ITEM	CALORIES	CARBS		FOOD ITEM	CALORIES	CARBS
TOTAL:				TOTAL:		

DATE _____

Exercise Activity: Hours ‖ Minutes ‖ Calories Burned

Measurements: Weight ‖ Chest ‖ Waist ‖ Hips

How Do I Feel About
My Progress Today?

BREAKFAST			LUNCH		
TIME:			TIME:		
LOCATION:			LOCATION:		
FOOD ITEM	CALORIES	CARBS	FOOD ITEM	CALORIES	CARBS
TOTAL:			TOTAL:		

DINNER			SNACK		
TIME:			TIME:		
LOCATION:			LOCATION:		
FOOD ITEM	CALORIES	CARBS	FOOD ITEM	CALORIES	CARBS
TOTAL:			TOTAL:		

DATE _____

Exercise Activity: Hours ‖ Minutes ‖ Calories Burned

Measurements: Weight ‖ Chest ‖ Waist ‖ Hips

How Do I Feel About
My Progress Today?

BREAKFAST			LUNCH		
TIME:			TIME:		
LOCATION:			LOCATION:		
FOOD ITEM	CALORIES	CARBS	FOOD ITEM	CALORIES	CARBS
TOTAL:			TOTAL:		

DINNER			SNACK		
TIME:			TIME:		
LOCATION:			LOCATION:		
FOOD ITEM	CALORIES	CARBS	FOOD ITEM	CALORIES	CARBS
TOTAL:			TOTAL:		

DATE _____

Exercise Activity: Hours || Minutes || Calories Burned

Measurements: Weight || Chest || Waist || Hips

How Do I Feel About
My Progress Today?

BREAKFAST			LUNCH		
TIME:			TIME:		
LOCATION:			LOCATION:		
FOOD ITEM	CALORIES	CARBS	FOOD ITEM	CALORIES	CARBS
TOTAL:			TOTAL:		

DINNER			SNACK		
TIME:			TIME:		
LOCATION:			LOCATION:		
FOOD ITEM	CALORIES	CARBS	FOOD ITEM	CALORIES	CARBS
TOTAL:			TOTAL:		

DATE _____

Exercise Activity: Hours || Minutes || Calories Burned

Measurements: Weight || Chest || Waist || Hips

How Do I Feel About My Progress Today?

BREAKFAST		
TIME:		
LOCATION:		
FOOD ITEM	CALORIES	CARBS
TOTAL:		

LUNCH		
TIME:		
LOCATION:		
FOOD ITEM	CALORIES	CARBS
TOTAL:		

DINNER		
TIME:		
LOCATION:		
FOOD ITEM	CALORIES	CARBS
TOTAL:		

SNACK		
TIME:		
LOCATION:		
FOOD ITEM	CALORIES	CARBS
TOTAL:		

DATE _____

Exercise Activity: Hours ‖ Minutes ‖ Calories Burned

Measurements: Weight ‖ Chest ‖ Waist ‖ Hips

How Do I Feel About My Progress Today?

BREAKFAST			LUNCH		
TIME:			TIME:		
LOCATION:			LOCATION:		
FOOD ITEM	CALORIES	CARBS	FOOD ITEM	CALORIES	CARBS
TOTAL:			TOTAL:		

DINNER			SNACK		
TIME:			TIME:		
LOCATION:			LOCATION:		
FOOD ITEM	CALORIES	CARBS	FOOD ITEM	CALORIES	CARBS
TOTAL:			TOTAL:		

Exercise Activity: Hours || Minutes || Calories Burned

Measurements: Weight || Chest || Waist || Hips

How Do I Feel About
My Progress Today?

BREAKFAST			**LUNCH**		
FOOD ITEM	CALORIES	CARBS	FOOD ITEM	CALORIES	CARBS
TOTAL:			TOTAL:		

TIME: (Breakfast) LOCATION: (Breakfast)
TIME: (Lunch) LOCATION: (Lunch)

DINNER			**SNACK**		
FOOD ITEM	CALORIES	CARBS	FOOD ITEM	CALORIES	CARBS
TOTAL:			TOTAL:		

TIME: (Dinner) LOCATION: (Dinner)
TIME: (Snack) LOCATION: (Snack)

Exercise Activity: Hours || Minutes || Calories Burned

Measurements: Weight || Chest || Waist || Hips

How Do I Feel About My Progress Today?

BREAKFAST			LUNCH		
TIME:			TIME:		
LOCATION:			LOCATION:		
FOOD ITEM	CALORIES	CARBS	FOOD ITEM	CALORIES	CARBS
TOTAL:			TOTAL:		

DINNER			SNACK		
TIME:			TIME:		
LOCATION:			LOCATION:		
FOOD ITEM	CALORIES	CARBS	FOOD ITEM	CALORIES	CARBS
TOTAL:			TOTAL:		

Exercise Activity: Hours || Minutes || Calories Burned

Measurements: Weight || Chest || Waist || Hips

How Do I Feel About
My Progress Today?

BREAKFAST				LUNCH			
TIME:				TIME:			
LOCATION:				LOCATION:			
FOOD ITEM		CALORIES	CARBS	FOOD ITEM		CALORIES	CARBS
TOTAL:				TOTAL:			

DINNER				SNACK			
TIME:				TIME:			
LOCATION:				LOCATION:			
FOOD ITEM		CALORIES	CARBS	FOOD ITEM		CALORIES	CARBS
TOTAL:				TOTAL:			

DATE _____

Exercise Activity: Hours || Minutes || Calories Burned

Measurements: Weight || Chest || Waist || Hips

How Do I Feel About
My Progress Today?

BREAKFAST			LUNCH		
TIME:			TIME:		
LOCATION:			LOCATION:		
FOOD ITEM	CALORIES	CARBS	FOOD ITEM	CALORIES	CARBS
TOTAL:			TOTAL:		

DINNER			SNACK		
TIME:			TIME:		
LOCATION:			LOCATION:		
FOOD ITEM	CALORIES	CARBS	FOOD ITEM	CALORIES	CARBS
TOTAL:			TOTAL:		

Exercise Activity: Hours || Minutes || Calories Burned

Measurements: Weight || Chest || Waist || Hips

How Do I Feel About
My Progress Today?

BREAKFAST			LUNCH		
TIME:			TIME:		
LOCATION:			LOCATION:		
FOOD ITEM	CALORIES	CARBS	FOOD ITEM	CALORIES	CARBS
TOTAL:			TOTAL:		
DINNER			**SNACK**		
TIME:			TIME:		
LOCATION:			LOCATION:		
FOOD ITEM	CALORIES	CARBS	FOOD ITEM	CALORIES	CARBS
TOTAL:			TOTAL:		

DATE _____

Exercise Activity: Hours ‖ Minutes ‖ Calories Burned

Measurements: Weight ‖ Chest ‖ Waist ‖ Hips

How Do I Feel About
My Progress Today?

BREAKFAST			LUNCH		
TIME:			TIME:		
LOCATION:			LOCATION:		
FOOD ITEM	CALORIES	CARBS	FOOD ITEM	CALORIES	CARBS
TOTAL:			TOTAL:		

DINNER			SNACK		
TIME:			TIME:		
LOCATION:			LOCATION:		
FOOD ITEM	CALORIES	CARBS	FOOD ITEM	CALORIES	CARBS
TOTAL:			TOTAL:		

DATE _____

Exercise Activity: Hours ‖ Minutes ‖ Calories Burned

Measurements: Weight ‖ Chest ‖ Waist ‖ Hips

How Do I Feel About
My Progress Today?

BREAKFAST				LUNCH			
TIME:				TIME:			
LOCATION:				LOCATION:			
FOOD ITEM		CALORIES	CARBS	FOOD ITEM		CALORIES	CARBS
TOTAL:				TOTAL:			

DINNER				SNACK			
TIME:				TIME:			
LOCATION:				LOCATION:			
FOOD ITEM		CALORIES	CARBS	FOOD ITEM		CALORIES	CARBS
TOTAL:				TOTAL:			

DATE _____

Exercise Activity: Hours ‖ Minutes ‖ Calories Burned

Measurements: Weight ‖ Chest ‖ Waist ‖ Hips

How Do I Feel About
My Progress Today?

BREAKFAST			LUNCH		
TIME:			TIME:		
LOCATION:			LOCATION:		
FOOD ITEM	CALORIES	CARBS	FOOD ITEM	CALORIES	CARBS
TOTAL:			TOTAL:		

DINNER			SNACK		
TIME:			TIME:		
LOCATION:			LOCATION:		
FOOD ITEM	CALORIES	CARBS	FOOD ITEM	CALORIES	CARBS
TOTAL:			TOTAL:		

DATE _____

Exercise Activity: Hours || Minutes || Calories Burned

_____

Measurements: Weight || Chest || Waist || Hips

_____

How Do I Feel About
My Progress Today?

BREAKFAST			LUNCH		
TIME:			TIME:		
LOCATION:			LOCATION:		
FOOD ITEM	CALORIES	CARBS	FOOD ITEM	CALORIES	CARBS
TOTAL:			TOTAL:		

DINNER			SNACK		
TIME:			TIME:		
LOCATION:			LOCATION:		
FOOD ITEM	CALORIES	CARBS	FOOD ITEM	CALORIES	CARBS
TOTAL:			TOTAL:		

DATE _____

Exercise Activity: Hours || Minutes || Calories Burned

Measurements: Weight || Chest || Waist || Hips

How Do I Feel About
My Progress Today?

BREAKFAST			LUNCH		
TIME:			TIME:		
LOCATION:			LOCATION:		
FOOD ITEM	CALORIES	CARBS	FOOD ITEM	CALORIES	CARBS
TOTAL:			TOTAL:		

DINNER			SNACK		
TIME:			TIME:		
LOCATION:			LOCATION:		
FOOD ITEM	CALORIES	CARBS	FOOD ITEM	CALORIES	CARBS
TOTAL:			TOTAL:		

Exercise Activity: Hours ‖ Minutes ‖ Calories Burned

Measurements: Weight ‖ Chest ‖ Waist ‖ Hips

How Do I Feel About
My Progress Today?

BREAKFAST			LUNCH		
TIME:			TIME:		
LOCATION:			LOCATION:		
FOOD ITEM	CALORIES	CARBS	FOOD ITEM	CALORIES	CARBS
TOTAL:			TOTAL:		

DINNER			SNACK		
TIME:			TIME:		
LOCATION:			LOCATION:		
FOOD ITEM	CALORIES	CARBS	FOOD ITEM	CALORIES	CARBS
TOTAL:			TOTAL:		

DATE _____

Exercise Activity: Hours || Minutes || Calories Burned

Measurements: Weight || Chest || Waist || Hips

How Do I Feel About My Progress Today?

BREAKFAST			LUNCH		
TIME:			TIME:		
LOCATION:			LOCATION:		
FOOD ITEM	CALORIES	CARBS	FOOD ITEM	CALORIES	CARBS
TOTAL:			TOTAL:		

DINNER			SNACK		
TIME:			TIME:		
LOCATION:			LOCATION:		
FOOD ITEM	CALORIES	CARBS	FOOD ITEM	CALORIES	CARBS
TOTAL:			TOTAL:		

DATE _____

Exercise Activity: Hours || Minutes || Calories Burned

Measurements: Weight || Chest || Waist || Hips

How Do I Feel About My Progress Today?

BREAKFAST			LUNCH		
TIME:			TIME:		
LOCATION:			LOCATION:		
FOOD ITEM	CALORIES	CARBS	FOOD ITEM	CALORIES	CARBS
TOTAL:			TOTAL:		

DINNER			SNACK		
TIME:			TIME:		
LOCATION:			LOCATION:		
FOOD ITEM	CALORIES	CARBS	FOOD ITEM	CALORIES	CARBS
TOTAL:			TOTAL:		

DATE _____

Exercise Activity: Hours || Minutes || Calories Burned

Measurements: Weight || Chest || Waist || Hips

How Do I Feel About
My Progress Today?

BREAKFAST			LUNCH		
TIME:			TIME:		
LOCATION:			LOCATION:		
FOOD ITEM	CALORIES	CARBS	FOOD ITEM	CALORIES	CARBS
TOTAL:			TOTAL:		

DINNER			SNACK		
TIME:			TIME:		
LOCATION:			LOCATION:		
FOOD ITEM	CALORIES	CARBS	FOOD ITEM	CALORIES	CARBS
TOTAL:			TOTAL:		

Exercise Activity: Hours || Minutes || Calories Burned

_____

Measurements: Weight || Chest || Waist || Hips

_____

How Do I Feel About
My Progress Today?

BREAKFAST			LUNCH		
TIME:			TIME:		
LOCATION:			LOCATION:		
FOOD ITEM	CALORIES	CARBS	FOOD ITEM	CALORIES	CARBS
TOTAL:			TOTAL:		

DINNER			SNACK		
TIME:			TIME:		
LOCATION:			LOCATION:		
FOOD ITEM	CALORIES	CARBS	FOOD ITEM	CALORIES	CARBS
TOTAL:			TOTAL:		

DATE _____

Exercise Activity: Hours || Minutes || Calories Burned

Measurements: Weight || Chest || Waist || Hips

How Do I Feel About
My Progress Today?

BREAKFAST			LUNCH		
TIME:			TIME:		
LOCATION:			LOCATION:		
FOOD ITEM	CALORIES	CARBS	FOOD ITEM	CALORIES	CARBS
TOTAL:			TOTAL:		

DINNER			SNACK		
TIME:			TIME:		
LOCATION:			LOCATION:		
FOOD ITEM	CALORIES	CARBS	FOOD ITEM	CALORIES	CARBS
TOTAL:			TOTAL:		

Exercise Activity: Hours || Minutes || Calories Burned

Measurements: Weight || Chest || Waist || Hips

How Do I Feel About
My Progress Today?

BREAKFAST			LUNCH		
TIME:			TIME:		
LOCATION:			LOCATION:		
FOOD ITEM	CALORIES	CARBS	FOOD ITEM	CALORIES	CARBS
TOTAL:			TOTAL:		
DINNER			SNACK		
TIME:			TIME:		
LOCATION:			LOCATION:		
FOOD ITEM	CALORIES	CARBS	FOOD ITEM	CALORIES	CARBS
TOTAL:			TOTAL:		

DATE _____

Exercise Activity: Hours || Minutes || Calories Burned

Measurements: Weight || Chest || Waist || Hips

How Do I Feel About
My Progress Today?

BREAKFAST			LUNCH		
TIME:			TIME:		
LOCATION:			LOCATION:		
FOOD ITEM	CALORIES	CARBS	FOOD ITEM	CALORIES	CARBS
TOTAL:			TOTAL:		

DINNER			SNACK		
TIME:			TIME:		
LOCATION:			LOCATION:		
FOOD ITEM	CALORIES	CARBS	FOOD ITEM	CALORIES	CARBS
TOTAL:			TOTAL:		

DATE _____

Exercise Activity: Hours || Minutes || Calories Burned

Measurements: Weight || Chest || Waist || Hips

How Do I Feel About
My Progress Today?

BREAKFAST			LUNCH		
TIME:			TIME:		
LOCATION:			LOCATION:		
FOOD ITEM	CALORIES	CARBS	FOOD ITEM	CALORIES	CARBS
TOTAL:			TOTAL:		

DINNER			SNACK		
TIME:			TIME:		
LOCATION:			LOCATION:		
FOOD ITEM	CALORIES	CARBS	FOOD ITEM	CALORIES	CARBS
TOTAL:			TOTAL:		

DATE _____

Exercise Activity: Hours || Minutes || Calories Burned

_____

Measurements: Weight || Chest || Waist || Hips

_____

How Do I Feel About
My Progress Today?

BREAKFAST			LUNCH		
TIME:			TIME:		
LOCATION:			LOCATION:		
FOOD ITEM	CALORIES	CARBS	FOOD ITEM	CALORIES	CARBS
TOTAL:			TOTAL:		

DINNER			SNACK		
TIME:			TIME:		
LOCATION:			LOCATION:		
FOOD ITEM	CALORIES	CARBS	FOOD ITEM	CALORIES	CARBS
TOTAL:			TOTAL:		

Exercise Activity: Hours || Minutes || Calories Burned

Measurements: Weight || Chest || Waist || Hips

How Do I Feel About
My Progress Today?

BREAKFAST			LUNCH		
TIME:			TIME:		
LOCATION:			LOCATION:		
FOOD ITEM	CALORIES	CARBS	FOOD ITEM	CALORIES	CARBS
TOTAL:			TOTAL:		

DINNER			SNACK		
TIME:			TIME:		
LOCATION:			LOCATION:		
FOOD ITEM	CALORIES	CARBS	FOOD ITEM	CALORIES	CARBS
TOTAL:			TOTAL:		

DATE _____

Exercise Activity: Hours ‖ Minutes ‖ Calories Burned

Measurements: Weight ‖ Chest ‖ Waist ‖ Hips

How Do I Feel About
My Progress Today?

BREAKFAST			LUNCH		
TIME:			TIME:		
LOCATION:			LOCATION:		
FOOD ITEM	CALORIES	CARBS	FOOD ITEM	CALORIES	CARBS
TOTAL:			TOTAL:		

DINNER			SNACK		
TIME:			TIME:		
LOCATION:			LOCATION:		
FOOD ITEM	CALORIES	CARBS	FOOD ITEM	CALORIES	CARBS
TOTAL:			TOTAL:		

DATE _____

Exercise Activity: Hours || Minutes || Calories Burned

Measurements: Weight || Chest || Waist || Hips

How Do I Feel About
My Progress Today?

BREAKFAST			LUNCH		
TIME:			TIME:		
LOCATION:			LOCATION:		
FOOD ITEM	CALORIES	CARBS	FOOD ITEM	CALORIES	CARBS
TOTAL:			TOTAL:		

DINNER			SNACK		
TIME:			TIME:		
LOCATION:			LOCATION:		
FOOD ITEM	CALORIES	CARBS	FOOD ITEM	CALORIES	CARBS
TOTAL:			TOTAL:		

DATE _____

Exercise Activity: Hours || Minutes || Calories Burned

Measurements: Weight || Chest || Waist || Hips

How Do I Feel About My Progress Today?

BREAKFAST			LUNCH		
TIME:			TIME:		
LOCATION:			LOCATION:		
FOOD ITEM	CALORIES	CARBS	FOOD ITEM	CALORIES	CARBS
TOTAL:			TOTAL:		

DINNER			SNACK		
TIME:			TIME:		
LOCATION:			LOCATION:		
FOOD ITEM	CALORIES	CARBS	FOOD ITEM	CALORIES	CARBS
TOTAL:			TOTAL:		

Exercise Activity: Hours || Minutes || Calories Burned

Measurements: Weight || Chest || Waist || Hips

How Do I Feel About
My Progress Today?

BREAKFAST			LUNCH		
TIME:			TIME:		
LOCATION:			LOCATION:		
FOOD ITEM	CALORIES	CARBS	FOOD ITEM	CALORIES	CARBS
TOTAL:			TOTAL:		

DINNER			SNACK		
TIME:			TIME:		
LOCATION:			LOCATION:		
FOOD ITEM	CALORIES	CARBS	FOOD ITEM	CALORIES	CARBS
TOTAL:			TOTAL:		

Exercise Activity: Hours ‖ Minutes ‖ Calories Burned

Measurements: Weight ‖ Chest ‖ Waist ‖ Hips

How Do I Feel About My Progress Today?

BREAKFAST			LUNCH		
TIME:			TIME:		
LOCATION:			LOCATION:		
FOOD ITEM	CALORIES	CARBS	FOOD ITEM	CALORIES	CARBS
TOTAL:			TOTAL:		

DINNER			SNACK		
TIME:			TIME:		
LOCATION:			LOCATION:		
FOOD ITEM	CALORIES	CARBS	FOOD ITEM	CALORIES	CARBS
TOTAL:			TOTAL:		

Exercise Activity: Hours ‖ Minutes ‖ Calories Burned

Measurements: Weight ‖ Chest ‖ Waist ‖ Hips

How Do I Feel About
My Progress Today?

BREAKFAST		
TIME:		
LOCATION:		
FOOD ITEM	CALORIES	CARBS
TOTAL:		

LUNCH		
TIME:		
LOCATION:		
FOOD ITEM	CALORIES	CARBS
TOTAL:		

DINNER		
TIME:		
LOCATION:		
FOOD ITEM	CALORIES	CARBS
TOTAL:		

SNACK		
TIME:		
LOCATION:		
FOOD ITEM	CALORIES	CARBS
TOTAL:		

Exercise Activity: Hours || Minutes || Calories Burned

Measurements: Weight || Chest || Waist || Hips

How Do I Feel About
My Progress Today?

BREAKFAST			LUNCH		
TIME:			TIME:		
LOCATION:			LOCATION:		
FOOD ITEM	CALORIES	CARBS	FOOD ITEM	CALORIES	CARBS
TOTAL:			TOTAL:		

DINNER			SNACK		
TIME:			TIME:		
LOCATION:			LOCATION:		
FOOD ITEM	CALORIES	CARBS	FOOD ITEM	CALORIES	CARBS
TOTAL:			TOTAL:		

Exercise Activity: Hours ‖ Minutes ‖ Calories Burned

Measurements: Weight ‖ Chest ‖ Waist ‖ Hips

How Do I Feel About
My Progress Today?

BREAKFAST			LUNCH		
TIME:			TIME:		
LOCATION:			LOCATION:		
FOOD ITEM	CALORIES	CARBS	FOOD ITEM	CALORIES	CARBS
TOTAL:			TOTAL:		

DINNER			SNACK		
TIME:			TIME:		
LOCATION:			LOCATION:		
FOOD ITEM	CALORIES	CARBS	FOOD ITEM	CALORIES	CARBS
TOTAL:			TOTAL:		

DATE _____

Exercise Activity: Hours || Minutes || Calories Burned

Measurements: Weight || Chest || Waist || Hips

How Do I Feel About
My Progress Today?

BREAKFAST			**LUNCH**		
TIME:			TIME:		
LOCATION:			LOCATION:		
FOOD ITEM	CALORIES	CARBS	FOOD ITEM	CALORIES	CARBS
TOTAL:			TOTAL:		
DINNER			**SNACK**		
TIME:			TIME:		
LOCATION:			LOCATION:		
FOOD ITEM	CALORIES	CARBS	FOOD ITEM	CALORIES	CARBS
TOTAL:			TOTAL:		

Exercise Activity: Hours || Minutes || Calories Burned

Measurements: Weight || Chest || Waist || Hips

How Do I Feel About
My Progress Today?

BREAKFAST			LUNCH		
TIME:			TIME:		
LOCATION:			LOCATION:		
FOOD ITEM	CALORIES	CARBS	FOOD ITEM	CALORIES	CARBS
TOTAL:			TOTAL:		

DINNER			SNACK		
TIME:			TIME:		
LOCATION:			LOCATION:		
FOOD ITEM	CALORIES	CARBS	FOOD ITEM	CALORIES	CARBS
TOTAL:			TOTAL:		

DATE _____

Exercise Activity: Hours || Minutes || Calories Burned

Measurements: Weight || Chest || Waist || Hips

How Do I Feel About
My Progress Today?

BREAKFAST			LUNCH		
TIME:			TIME:		
LOCATION:			LOCATION:		
FOOD ITEM	CALORIES	CARBS	FOOD ITEM	CALORIES	CARBS
TOTAL:			TOTAL:		

DINNER			SNACK		
TIME:			TIME:		
LOCATION:			LOCATION:		
FOOD ITEM	CALORIES	CARBS	FOOD ITEM	CALORIES	CARBS
TOTAL:			TOTAL:		

DATE _____

Exercise Activity: Hours || Minutes || Calories Burned

Measurements: Weight || Chest || Waist || Hips

How Do I Feel About
My Progress Today?

BREAKFAST			LUNCH		
TIME:			TIME:		
LOCATION:			LOCATION:		
FOOD ITEM	CALORIES	CARBS	FOOD ITEM	CALORIES	CARBS
TOTAL:			TOTAL:		

DINNER			SNACK		
TIME:			TIME:		
LOCATION:			LOCATION:		
FOOD ITEM	CALORIES	CARBS	FOOD ITEM	CALORIES	CARBS
TOTAL:			TOTAL:		

Exercise Activity: Hours ‖ Minutes ‖ Calories Burned

Measurements: Weight ‖ Chest ‖ Waist ‖ Hips

How Do I Feel About My Progress Today?

BREAKFAST			LUNCH		
TIME:			TIME:		
LOCATION:			LOCATION:		
FOOD ITEM	CALORIES	CARBS	FOOD ITEM	CALORIES	CARBS
TOTAL:			TOTAL:		

DINNER			SNACK		
TIME:			TIME:		
LOCATION:			LOCATION:		
FOOD ITEM	CALORIES	CARBS	FOOD ITEM	CALORIES	CARBS
TOTAL:			TOTAL:		

DATE _____

Exercise Activity: Hours || Minutes || Calories Burned

_____

Measurements: Weight || Chest || Waist || Hips

_____

How Do I Feel About
My Progress Today?

BREAKFAST			LUNCH		
TIME:			TIME:		
LOCATION:			LOCATION:		
FOOD ITEM	CALORIES	CARBS	FOOD ITEM	CALORIES	CARBS
TOTAL:			TOTAL:		

DINNER			SNACK		
TIME:			TIME:		
LOCATION:			LOCATION:		
FOOD ITEM	CALORIES	CARBS	FOOD ITEM	CALORIES	CARBS
TOTAL:			TOTAL:		

DATE _____

Exercise Activity: Hours || Minutes || Calories Burned

Measurements: Weight || Chest || Waist || Hips

How Do I Feel About My Progress Today?

BREAKFAST			LUNCH		
TIME:			TIME:		
LOCATION:			LOCATION:		
FOOD ITEM	CALORIES	CARBS	FOOD ITEM	CALORIES	CARBS
TOTAL:			TOTAL:		

DINNER			SNACK		
TIME:			TIME:		
LOCATION:			LOCATION:		
FOOD ITEM	CALORIES	CARBS	FOOD ITEM	CALORIES	CARBS
TOTAL:			TOTAL:		

DATE _____

Exercise Activity: Hours ‖ Minutes ‖ Calories Burned

Measurements: Weight ‖ Chest ‖ Waist ‖ Hips

How Do I Feel About
My Progress Today?

BREAKFAST				LUNCH		
TIME:				TIME:		
LOCATION:				LOCATION:		
FOOD ITEM		CALORIES	CARBS	FOOD ITEM		CALORIES	CARBS
TOTAL:				TOTAL:		

DINNER				SNACK		
TIME:				TIME:		
LOCATION:				LOCATION:		
FOOD ITEM		CALORIES	CARBS	FOOD ITEM		CALORIES	CARBS
TOTAL:				TOTAL:		

DATE _____

Exercise Activity: Hours || Minutes || Calories Burned

_____

Measurements: Weight || Chest || Waist || Hips

_____

How Do I Feel About
My Progress Today?

BREAKFAST			LUNCH		
TIME:			TIME:		
LOCATION:			LOCATION:		
FOOD ITEM	CALORIES	CARBS	FOOD ITEM	CALORIES	CARBS
TOTAL:			TOTAL:		

DINNER			SNACK		
TIME:			TIME:		
LOCATION:			LOCATION:		
FOOD ITEM	CALORIES	CARBS	FOOD ITEM	CALORIES	CARBS
TOTAL:			TOTAL:		

DATE _____

Exercise Activity: Hours ‖ Minutes ‖ Calories Burned

Measurements: Weight ‖ Chest ‖ Waist ‖ Hips

How Do I Feel About
My Progress Today?

BREAKFAST			LUNCH		
TIME:			TIME:		
LOCATION:			LOCATION:		
FOOD ITEM	CALORIES	CARBS	FOOD ITEM	CALORIES	CARBS
TOTAL:			TOTAL:		

DINNER			SNACK		
TIME:			TIME:		
LOCATION:			LOCATION:		
FOOD ITEM	CALORIES	CARBS	FOOD ITEM	CALORIES	CARBS
TOTAL:			TOTAL:		

Exercise Activity: Hours || Minutes || Calories Burned

Measurements: Weight || Chest || Waist || Hips

How Do I Feel About
My Progress Today?

BREAKFAST			LUNCH		
TIME:			TIME:		
LOCATION:			LOCATION:		
FOOD ITEM	CALORIES	CARBS	FOOD ITEM	CALORIES	CARBS
TOTAL:			TOTAL:		

DINNER			SNACK		
TIME:			TIME:		
LOCATION:			LOCATION:		
FOOD ITEM	CALORIES	CARBS	FOOD ITEM	CALORIES	CARBS
TOTAL:			TOTAL:		

Exercise Activity: Hours || Minutes || Calories Burned

Measurements: Weight || Chest || Waist || Hips

How Do I Feel About My Progress Today?

BREAKFAST			LUNCH		
TIME:			TIME:		
LOCATION:			LOCATION:		
FOOD ITEM	CALORIES	CARBS	FOOD ITEM	CALORIES	CARBS
TOTAL:			TOTAL:		

DINNER			SNACK		
TIME:			TIME:		
LOCATION:			LOCATION:		
FOOD ITEM	CALORIES	CARBS	FOOD ITEM	CALORIES	CARBS
TOTAL:			TOTAL:		

DATE _____

Exercise Activity: Hours || Minutes || Calories Burned

Measurements: Weight || Chest || Waist || Hips

How Do I Feel About
My Progress Today?

BREAKFAST			LUNCH		
TIME:			TIME:		
LOCATION:			LOCATION:		
FOOD ITEM	CALORIES	CARBS	FOOD ITEM	CALORIES	CARBS
TOTAL:			TOTAL:		

DINNER			SNACK		
TIME:			TIME:		
LOCATION:			LOCATION:		
FOOD ITEM	CALORIES	CARBS	FOOD ITEM	CALORIES	CARBS
TOTAL:			TOTAL:		

DATE _____

Exercise Activity: Hours || Minutes || Calories Burned

Measurements: Weight || Chest || Waist || Hips

How Do I Feel About
My Progress Today?

BREAKFAST			LUNCH		
TIME:			TIME:		
LOCATION:			LOCATION:		
FOOD ITEM	CALORIES	CARBS	FOOD ITEM	CALORIES	CARBS
TOTAL:			TOTAL:		

DINNER			SNACK		
TIME:			TIME:		
LOCATION:			LOCATION:		
FOOD ITEM	CALORIES	CARBS	FOOD ITEM	CALORIES	CARBS
TOTAL:			TOTAL:		

Exercise Activity: Hours || Minutes || Calories Burned

Measurements: Weight || Chest || Waist || Hips

How Do I Feel About
My Progress Today?

BREAKFAST			LUNCH		
TIME:			TIME:		
LOCATION:			LOCATION:		
FOOD ITEM	CALORIES	CARBS	FOOD ITEM	CALORIES	CARBS
TOTAL:			TOTAL:		

DINNER			SNACK		
TIME:			TIME:		
LOCATION:			LOCATION:		
FOOD ITEM	CALORIES	CARBS	FOOD ITEM	CALORIES	CARBS
TOTAL:			TOTAL:		

Exercise Activity: Hours ‖ Minutes ‖ Calories Burned

Measurements: Weight ‖ Chest ‖ Waist ‖ Hips

How Do I Feel About
My Progress Today?

BREAKFAST			**LUNCH**		
TIME:			TIME:		
LOCATION:			LOCATION:		
FOOD ITEM	CALORIES	CARBS	FOOD ITEM	CALORIES	CARBS
TOTAL:			TOTAL:		
DINNER			**SNACK**		
TIME:			TIME:		
LOCATION:			LOCATION:		
FOOD ITEM	CALORIES	CARBS	FOOD ITEM	CALORIES	CARBS
TOTAL:			TOTAL:		

Exercise Activity: Hours || Minutes || Calories Burned

Measurements: Weight || Chest || Waist || Hips

How Do I Feel About
My Progress Today?

BREAKFAST			LUNCH		
TIME:			TIME:		
LOCATION:			LOCATION:		
FOOD ITEM	CALORIES	CARBS	FOOD ITEM	CALORIES	CARBS
TOTAL:			TOTAL:		

DINNER			SNACK		
TIME:			TIME:		
LOCATION:			LOCATION:		
FOOD ITEM	CALORIES	CARBS	FOOD ITEM	CALORIES	CARBS
TOTAL:			TOTAL:		

Exercise Activity: Hours || Minutes || Calories Burned

Measurements: Weight || Chest || Waist || Hips

How Do I Feel About
My Progress Today?

BREAKFAST			LUNCH		
TIME:			TIME:		
LOCATION:			LOCATION:		
FOOD ITEM	CALORIES	CARBS	FOOD ITEM	CALORIES	CARBS
TOTAL:			TOTAL:		

DINNER			SNACK		
TIME:			TIME:		
LOCATION:			LOCATION:		
FOOD ITEM	CALORIES	CARBS	FOOD ITEM	CALORIES	CARBS
TOTAL:			TOTAL:		

DATE _____

Exercise Activity: Hours || Minutes || Calories Burned

Measurements: Weight || Chest || Waist || Hips

How Do I Feel About
My Progress Today?

BREAKFAST			LUNCH		
TIME:			TIME:		
LOCATION:			LOCATION:		
FOOD ITEM	CALORIES	CARBS	FOOD ITEM	CALORIES	CARBS
TOTAL:			TOTAL:		

DINNER			SNACK		
TIME:			TIME:		
LOCATION:			LOCATION:		
FOOD ITEM	CALORIES	CARBS	FOOD ITEM	CALORIES	CARBS
TOTAL:			TOTAL:		

DATE _____

Exercise Activity: Hours || Minutes || Calories Burned

Measurements: Weight || Chest || Waist || Hips

How Do I Feel About
My Progress Today?

BREAKFAST				LUNCH		
TIME:				TIME:		
LOCATION:				LOCATION:		
FOOD ITEM		CALORIES	CARBS	FOOD ITEM		CALORIES	CARBS
TOTAL:				TOTAL:		

DINNER				SNACK		
TIME:				TIME:		
LOCATION:				LOCATION:		
FOOD ITEM		CALORIES	CARBS	FOOD ITEM		CALORIES	CARBS
TOTAL:				TOTAL:		

DATE _____

Exercise Activity: Hours || Minutes || Calories Burned

Measurements: Weight || Chest || Waist || Hips

How Do I Feel About
My Progress Today?

BREAKFAST			LUNCH		
TIME:			TIME:		
LOCATION:			LOCATION:		
FOOD ITEM	CALORIES	CARBS	FOOD ITEM	CALORIES	CARBS
TOTAL:			TOTAL:		

DINNER			SNACK		
TIME:			TIME:		
LOCATION:			LOCATION:		
FOOD ITEM	CALORIES	CARBS	FOOD ITEM	CALORIES	CARBS
TOTAL:			TOTAL:		

DATE _____

Exercise Activity: Hours ‖ Minutes ‖ Calories Burned

Measurements: Weight ‖ Chest ‖ Waist ‖ Hips

How Do I Feel About
My Progress Today?

BREAKFAST			LUNCH		
TIME:			TIME:		
LOCATION:			LOCATION:		
FOOD ITEM	CALORIES	CARBS	FOOD ITEM	CALORIES	CARBS
TOTAL:			TOTAL:		

DINNER			SNACK		
TIME:			TIME:		
LOCATION:			LOCATION:		
FOOD ITEM	CALORIES	CARBS	FOOD ITEM	CALORIES	CARBS
TOTAL:			TOTAL:		

DATE _____

Exercise Activity: Hours || Minutes || Calories Burned

Measurements: Weight || Chest || Waist || Hips

How Do I Feel About
My Progress Today?

BREAKFAST				LUNCH		
TIME:				TIME:		
LOCATION:				LOCATION:		
FOOD ITEM		CALORIES	CARBS	FOOD ITEM		CALORIES	CARBS
TOTAL:				TOTAL:		

DINNER				SNACK		
TIME:				TIME:		
LOCATION:				LOCATION:		
FOOD ITEM		CALORIES	CARBS	FOOD ITEM		CALORIES	CARBS
TOTAL:				TOTAL:		

DATE _____

Exercise Activity: Hours || Minutes || Calories Burned

Measurements: Weight || Chest || Waist || Hips

How Do I Feel About
My Progress Today?

BREAKFAST			LUNCH		
TIME:			TIME:		
LOCATION:			LOCATION:		
FOOD ITEM	CALORIES	CARBS	FOOD ITEM	CALORIES	CARBS
TOTAL:			TOTAL:		

DINNER			SNACK		
TIME:			TIME:		
LOCATION:			LOCATION:		
FOOD ITEM	CALORIES	CARBS	FOOD ITEM	CALORIES	CARBS
TOTAL:			TOTAL:		

DATE _____

Exercise Activity: Hours || Minutes || Calories Burned

Measurements: Weight || Chest || Waist || Hips

How Do I Feel About
My Progress Today?

BREAKFAST			LUNCH		
TIME:			TIME:		
LOCATION:			LOCATION:		
FOOD ITEM	CALORIES	CARBS	FOOD ITEM	CALORIES	CARBS
TOTAL:			TOTAL:		

DINNER			SNACK		
TIME:			TIME:		
LOCATION:			LOCATION:		
FOOD ITEM	CALORIES	CARBS	FOOD ITEM	CALORIES	CARBS
TOTAL:			TOTAL:		

DATE _____

Exercise Activity: Hours ‖ Minutes ‖ Calories Burned

Measurements: Weight ‖ Chest ‖ Waist ‖ Hips

How Do I Feel About
My Progress Today?

BREAKFAST			LUNCH		
TIME:			TIME:		
LOCATION:			LOCATION:		
FOOD ITEM	CALORIES	CARBS	FOOD ITEM	CALORIES	CARBS
TOTAL:			TOTAL:		

DINNER			SNACK		
TIME:			TIME:		
LOCATION:			LOCATION:		
FOOD ITEM	CALORIES	CARBS	FOOD ITEM	CALORIES	CARBS
TOTAL:			TOTAL:		

Exercise Activity: Hours || Minutes || Calories Burned

Measurements: Weight || Chest || Waist || Hips

How Do I Feel About
My Progress Today?

BREAKFAST			LUNCH		
TIME:			TIME:		
LOCATION:			LOCATION:		
FOOD ITEM	CALORIES	CARBS	FOOD ITEM	CALORIES	CARBS
TOTAL:			TOTAL:		

DINNER			SNACK		
TIME:			TIME:		
LOCATION:			LOCATION:		
FOOD ITEM	CALORIES	CARBS	FOOD ITEM	CALORIES	CARBS
TOTAL:			TOTAL:		

DATE _____

Exercise Activity: Hours || Minutes || Calories Burned

_____

Measurements: Weight || Chest || Waist || Hips

_____

How Do I Feel About
My Progress Today?

BREAKFAST			LUNCH		
TIME:			TIME:		
LOCATION:			LOCATION:		
FOOD ITEM	CALORIES	CARBS	FOOD ITEM	CALORIES	CARBS
TOTAL:			TOTAL:		

DINNER			SNACK		
TIME:			TIME:		
LOCATION:			LOCATION:		
FOOD ITEM	CALORIES	CARBS	FOOD ITEM	CALORIES	CARBS
TOTAL:			TOTAL:		

Exercise Activity: Hours || Minutes || Calories Burned

Measurements: Weight || Chest || Waist || Hips

How Do I Feel About
My Progress Today?

BREAKFAST			LUNCH		
TIME:			TIME:		
LOCATION:			LOCATION:		
FOOD ITEM	CALORIES	CARBS	FOOD ITEM	CALORIES	CARBS
TOTAL:			TOTAL:		

DINNER			SNACK		
TIME:			TIME:		
LOCATION:			LOCATION:		
FOOD ITEM	CALORIES	CARBS	FOOD ITEM	CALORIES	CARBS
TOTAL:			TOTAL:		

Exercise Activity: Hours || Minutes || Calories Burned

Measurements: Weight || Chest || Waist || Hips

How Do I Feel About
My Progress Today?

BREAKFAST			LUNCH		
TIME:			TIME:		
LOCATION:			LOCATION:		
FOOD ITEM	CALORIES	CARBS	FOOD ITEM	CALORIES	CARBS
TOTAL:			TOTAL:		

DINNER			SNACK		
TIME:			TIME:		
LOCATION:			LOCATION:		
FOOD ITEM	CALORIES	CARBS	FOOD ITEM	CALORIES	CARBS
TOTAL:			TOTAL:		

Exercise Activity: Hours ‖ Minutes ‖ Calories Burned

Measurements: Weight ‖ Chest ‖ Waist ‖ Hips

How Do I Feel About My Progress Today?

BREAKFAST			**LUNCH**		
TIME:			TIME:		
LOCATION:			LOCATION:		
FOOD ITEM	CALORIES	CARBS	FOOD ITEM	CALORIES	CARBS
TOTAL:			TOTAL:		

DINNER			**SNACK**		
TIME:			TIME:		
LOCATION:			LOCATION:		
FOOD ITEM	CALORIES	CARBS	FOOD ITEM	CALORIES	CARBS
TOTAL:			TOTAL:		

DATE _____

Exercise Activity: Hours || Minutes || Calories Burned

Measurements: Weight || Chest || Waist || Hips

How Do I Feel About
My Progress Today?

BREAKFAST				LUNCH		
TIME:				TIME:		
LOCATION:				LOCATION:		
FOOD ITEM	CALORIES	CARBS		FOOD ITEM	CALORIES	CARBS
TOTAL:				TOTAL:		

DINNER				SNACK		
TIME:				TIME:		
LOCATION:				LOCATION:		
FOOD ITEM	CALORIES	CARBS		FOOD ITEM	CALORIES	CARBS
TOTAL:				TOTAL:		

DATE _____

Exercise Activity: Hours || Minutes || Calories Burned

_____

Measurements: Weight || Chest || Waist || Hips

_____

How Do I Feel About
My Progress Today?

BREAKFAST			LUNCH		
TIME:			TIME:		
LOCATION:			LOCATION:		
FOOD ITEM	CALORIES	CARBS	FOOD ITEM	CALORIES	CARBS
TOTAL:			TOTAL:		

DINNER			SNACK		
TIME:			TIME:		
LOCATION:			LOCATION:		
FOOD ITEM	CALORIES	CARBS	FOOD ITEM	CALORIES	CARBS
TOTAL:			TOTAL:		

Exercise Activity: Hours || Minutes || Calories Burned

Measurements: Weight || Chest || Waist || Hips

How Do I Feel About
My Progress Today?

BREAKFAST			LUNCH		
TIME:			TIME:		
LOCATION:			LOCATION:		
FOOD ITEM	CALORIES	CARBS	FOOD ITEM	CALORIES	CARBS
TOTAL:			TOTAL:		

DINNER			SNACK		
TIME:			TIME:		
LOCATION:			LOCATION:		
FOOD ITEM	CALORIES	CARBS	FOOD ITEM	CALORIES	CARBS
TOTAL:			TOTAL:		

Exercise Activity: Hours ‖ Minutes ‖ Calories Burned

Measurements: Weight ‖ Chest ‖ Waist ‖ Hips

How Do I Feel About
My Progress Today?

BREAKFAST			LUNCH		
TIME:			TIME:		
LOCATION:			LOCATION:		
FOOD ITEM	CALORIES	CARBS	FOOD ITEM	CALORIES	CARBS
TOTAL:			TOTAL:		

DINNER			SNACK		
TIME:			TIME:		
LOCATION:			LOCATION:		
FOOD ITEM	CALORIES	CARBS	FOOD ITEM	CALORIES	CARBS
TOTAL:			TOTAL:		

Exercise Activity: Hours || Minutes || Calories Burned

Measurements: Weight || Chest || Waist || Hips

How Do I Feel About
My Progress Today?

BREAKFAST			LUNCH		
TIME:			TIME:		
LOCATION:			LOCATION:		
FOOD ITEM	CALORIES	CARBS	FOOD ITEM	CALORIES	CARBS
TOTAL:			TOTAL:		

DINNER			SNACK		
TIME:			TIME:		
LOCATION:			LOCATION:		
FOOD ITEM	CALORIES	CARBS	FOOD ITEM	CALORIES	CARBS
TOTAL:			TOTAL:		

Exercise Activity: Hours || Minutes || Calories Burned

Measurements: Weight || Chest || Waist || Hips

How Do I Feel About
My Progress Today?

BREAKFAST			LUNCH		
TIME:			TIME:		
LOCATION:			LOCATION:		
FOOD ITEM	CALORIES	CARBS	FOOD ITEM	CALORIES	CARBS
TOTAL:			TOTAL:		

DINNER			SNACK		
TIME:			TIME:		
LOCATION:			LOCATION:		
FOOD ITEM	CALORIES	CARBS	FOOD ITEM	CALORIES	CARBS
TOTAL:			TOTAL:		

Exercise Activity: Hours || Minutes || Calories Burned

Measurements: Weight || Chest || Waist || Hips

How Do I Feel About
My Progress Today?

BREAKFAST			LUNCH		
TIME:			TIME:		
LOCATION:			LOCATION:		
FOOD ITEM	CALORIES	CARBS	FOOD ITEM	CALORIES	CARBS
TOTAL:			TOTAL:		

DINNER			SNACK		
TIME:			TIME:		
LOCATION:			LOCATION:		
FOOD ITEM	CALORIES	CARBS	FOOD ITEM	CALORIES	CARBS
TOTAL:			TOTAL:		

DATE _____

Exercise Activity: Hours || Minutes || Calories Burned

_____

Measurements: Weight || Chest || Waist || Hips

_____

How Do I Feel About
My Progress Today?

BREAKFAST			LUNCH		
TIME:			TIME:		
LOCATION:			LOCATION:		
FOOD ITEM	CALORIES	CARBS	FOOD ITEM	CALORIES	CARBS
TOTAL:			TOTAL:		

DINNER			SNACK		
TIME:			TIME:		
LOCATION:			LOCATION:		
FOOD ITEM	CALORIES	CARBS	FOOD ITEM	CALORIES	CARBS
TOTAL:			TOTAL:		

DATE _____

Exercise Activity: Hours || Minutes || Calories Burned

Measurements: Weight || Chest || Waist || Hips

How Do I Feel About
My Progress Today?

BREAKFAST			LUNCH		
TIME:			TIME:		
LOCATION:			LOCATION:		
FOOD ITEM	CALORIES	CARBS	FOOD ITEM	CALORIES	CARBS
TOTAL:			TOTAL:		

DINNER			SNACK		
TIME:			TIME:		
LOCATION:			LOCATION:		
FOOD ITEM	CALORIES	CARBS	FOOD ITEM	CALORIES	CARBS
TOTAL:			TOTAL:		

Exercise Activity: Hours ‖ Minutes ‖ Calories Burned

Measurements: Weight ‖ Chest ‖ Waist ‖ Hips

How Do I Feel About
My Progress Today?

BREAKFAST			**LUNCH**		
TIME:			TIME:		
LOCATION:			LOCATION:		
FOOD ITEM	CALORIES	CARBS	FOOD ITEM	CALORIES	CARBS
TOTAL:			TOTAL:		
DINNER			**SNACK**		
TIME:			TIME:		
LOCATION:			LOCATION:		
FOOD ITEM	CALORIES	CARBS	FOOD ITEM	CALORIES	CARBS
TOTAL:			TOTAL:		

DATE _____

Exercise Activity: Hours || Minutes || Calories Burned

Measurements: Weight || Chest || Waist || Hips

How Do I Feel About My Progress Today?

BREAKFAST			LUNCH		
TIME:			TIME:		
LOCATION:			LOCATION:		
FOOD ITEM	CALORIES	CARBS	FOOD ITEM	CALORIES	CARBS
TOTAL:			TOTAL:		

DINNER			SNACK		
TIME:			TIME:		
LOCATION:			LOCATION:		
FOOD ITEM	CALORIES	CARBS	FOOD ITEM	CALORIES	CARBS
TOTAL:			TOTAL:		

DATE _____

Exercise Activity: Hours || Minutes || Calories Burned

Measurements: Weight || Chest || Waist || Hips

How Do I Feel About
My Progress Today?

BREAKFAST			LUNCH		
TIME:			TIME:		
LOCATION:			LOCATION:		
FOOD ITEM	CALORIES	CARBS	FOOD ITEM	CALORIES	CARBS
TOTAL:			TOTAL:		

DINNER			SNACK		
TIME:			TIME:		
LOCATION:			LOCATION:		
FOOD ITEM	CALORIES	CARBS	FOOD ITEM	CALORIES	CARBS
TOTAL:			TOTAL:		

Exercise Activity: Hours || Minutes || Calories Burned

Measurements: Weight || Chest || Waist || Hips

How Do I Feel About
My Progress Today?   😄   😉   🤭   😟   😫

BREAKFAST				LUNCH		
TIME:				TIME:		
LOCATION:				LOCATION:		
FOOD ITEM	CALORIES	CARBS		FOOD ITEM	CALORIES	CARBS
TOTAL:				TOTAL:		

DINNER				SNACK		
TIME:				TIME:		
LOCATION:				LOCATION:		
FOOD ITEM	CALORIES	CARBS		FOOD ITEM	CALORIES	CARBS
TOTAL:				TOTAL:		

DATE _____

Exercise Activity: Hours || Minutes || Calories Burned

_____

Measurements: Weight || Chest || Waist || Hips

_____

How Do I Feel About
My Progress Today?

BREAKFAST			LUNCH		
TIME:			TIME:		
LOCATION:			LOCATION:		
FOOD ITEM	CALORIES	CARBS	FOOD ITEM	CALORIES	CARBS
TOTAL:			TOTAL:		

DINNER			SNACK		
TIME:			TIME:		
LOCATION:			LOCATION:		
FOOD ITEM	CALORIES	CARBS	FOOD ITEM	CALORIES	CARBS
TOTAL:			TOTAL:		

Exercise Activity: Hours || Minutes || Calories Burned

_____

Measurements: Weight || Chest || Waist || Hips

_____

How Do I Feel About
My Progress Today?

BREAKFAST			**LUNCH**		
TIME:			TIME:		
LOCATION:			LOCATION:		
FOOD ITEM	CALORIES	CARBS	FOOD ITEM	CALORIES	CARBS
TOTAL:			TOTAL:		
DINNER			**SNACK**		
TIME:			TIME:		
LOCATION:			LOCATION:		
FOOD ITEM	CALORIES	CARBS	FOOD ITEM	CALORIES	CARBS
TOTAL:			TOTAL:		

DATE _____

Exercise Activity: Hours || Minutes || Calories Burned

Measurements: Weight || Chest || Waist || Hips

How Do I Feel About
My Progress Today?

BREAKFAST			LUNCH		
TIME:			TIME:		
LOCATION:			LOCATION:		
FOOD ITEM	CALORIES	CARBS	FOOD ITEM	CALORIES	CARBS
TOTAL:			TOTAL:		

DINNER			SNACK		
TIME:			TIME:		
LOCATION:			LOCATION:		
FOOD ITEM	CALORIES	CARBS	FOOD ITEM	CALORIES	CARBS
TOTAL:			TOTAL:		

DATE _____

Exercise Activity: Hours || Minutes || Calories Burned

Measurements: Weight || Chest || Waist || Hips

How Do I Feel About
My Progress Today?

BREAKFAST			LUNCH		
TIME:			TIME:		
LOCATION:			LOCATION:		
FOOD ITEM	CALORIES	CARBS	FOOD ITEM	CALORIES	CARBS
TOTAL:			TOTAL:		

DINNER			SNACK		
TIME:			TIME:		
LOCATION:			LOCATION:		
FOOD ITEM	CALORIES	CARBS	FOOD ITEM	CALORIES	CARBS
TOTAL:			TOTAL:		

DATE _____

Exercise Activity: Hours || Minutes || Calories Burned

Measurements: Weight || Chest || Waist || Hips

How Do I Feel About
My Progress Today?

BREAKFAST			LUNCH		
TIME:			TIME:		
LOCATION:			LOCATION:		
FOOD ITEM	CALORIES	CARBS	FOOD ITEM	CALORIES	CARBS
TOTAL:			TOTAL:		

DINNER			SNACK		
TIME:			TIME:		
LOCATION:			LOCATION:		
FOOD ITEM	CALORIES	CARBS	FOOD ITEM	CALORIES	CARBS
TOTAL:			TOTAL:		

DATE _____

Exercise Activity: Hours ‖ Minutes ‖ Calories Burned

Measurements: Weight ‖ Chest ‖ Waist ‖ Hips

How Do I Feel About
My Progress Today?

BREAKFAST				LUNCH			
TIME:				TIME:			
LOCATION:				LOCATION:			
FOOD ITEM		CALORIES	CARBS	FOOD ITEM		CALORIES	CARBS
TOTAL:				TOTAL:			

DINNER				SNACK			
TIME:				TIME:			
LOCATION:				LOCATION:			
FOOD ITEM		CALORIES	CARBS	FOOD ITEM		CALORIES	CARBS
TOTAL:				TOTAL:			

DATE _____

Exercise Activity: Hours || Minutes || Calories Burned

Measurements: Weight || Chest || Waist || Hips

How Do I Feel About
My Progress Today?

BREAKFAST			LUNCH		
TIME:			TIME:		
LOCATION:			LOCATION:		
FOOD ITEM	CALORIES	CARBS	FOOD ITEM	CALORIES	CARBS
TOTAL:			TOTAL:		

DINNER			SNACK		
TIME:			TIME:		
LOCATION:			LOCATION:		
FOOD ITEM	CALORIES	CARBS	FOOD ITEM	CALORIES	CARBS
TOTAL:			TOTAL:		

DATE _____

Exercise Activity: Hours || Minutes || Calories Burned

Measurements: Weight || Chest || Waist || Hips

How Do I Feel About
My Progress Today?

BREAKFAST			LUNCH		
TIME:			TIME:		
LOCATION:			LOCATION:		
FOOD ITEM	CALORIES	CARBS	FOOD ITEM	CALORIES	CARBS
TOTAL:			TOTAL:		

DINNER			SNACK		
TIME:			TIME:		
LOCATION:			LOCATION:		
FOOD ITEM	CALORIES	CARBS	FOOD ITEM	CALORIES	CARBS
TOTAL:			TOTAL:		

Exercise Activity: Hours ‖ Minutes ‖ Calories Burned

Measurements: Weight ‖ Chest ‖ Waist ‖ Hips

How Do I Feel About My Progress Today?

BREAKFAST			**LUNCH**		
TIME:			TIME:		
LOCATION:			LOCATION:		
FOOD ITEM	CALORIES	CARBS	FOOD ITEM	CALORIES	CARBS
TOTAL:			TOTAL:		

DINNER			**SNACK**		
TIME:			TIME:		
LOCATION:			LOCATION:		
FOOD ITEM	CALORIES	CARBS	FOOD ITEM	CALORIES	CARBS
TOTAL:			TOTAL:		

Exercise Activity: Hours || Minutes || Calories Burned

Measurements: Weight || Chest || Waist || Hips

How Do I Feel About
My Progress Today?

BREAKFAST			LUNCH		
TIME:			TIME:		
LOCATION:			LOCATION:		
FOOD ITEM	CALORIES	CARBS	FOOD ITEM	CALORIES	CARBS
TOTAL:			TOTAL:		

DINNER			SNACK		
TIME:			TIME:		
LOCATION:			LOCATION:		
FOOD ITEM	CALORIES	CARBS	FOOD ITEM	CALORIES	CARBS
TOTAL:			TOTAL:		

DATE _____

Exercise Activity: Hours ‖ Minutes ‖ Calories Burned

Measurements: Weight ‖ Chest ‖ Waist ‖ Hips

How Do I Feel About
My Progress Today?

BREAKFAST			LUNCH		
TIME:			TIME:		
LOCATION:			LOCATION:		
FOOD ITEM	CALORIES	CARBS	FOOD ITEM	CALORIES	CARBS
TOTAL:			TOTAL:		
DINNER			**SNACK**		
TIME:			TIME:		
LOCATION:			LOCATION:		
FOOD ITEM	CALORIES	CARBS	FOOD ITEM	CALORIES	CARBS
TOTAL:			TOTAL:		

Exercise Activity: Hours || Minutes || Calories Burned

Measurements: Weight || Chest || Waist || Hips

How Do I Feel About
My Progress Today?

BREAKFAST			LUNCH		
TIME:			TIME:		
LOCATION:			LOCATION:		
FOOD ITEM	CALORIES	CARBS	FOOD ITEM	CALORIES	CARBS
TOTAL:			TOTAL:		

DINNER			SNACK		
TIME:			TIME:		
LOCATION:			LOCATION:		
FOOD ITEM	CALORIES	CARBS	FOOD ITEM	CALORIES	CARBS
TOTAL:			TOTAL:		

Exercise Activity: Hours || Minutes || Calories Burned

Measurements: Weight || Chest || Waist || Hips

How Do I Feel About
My Progress Today?

BREAKFAST			LUNCH		
TIME:			TIME:		
LOCATION:			LOCATION:		
FOOD ITEM	CALORIES	CARBS	FOOD ITEM	CALORIES	CARBS
TOTAL:			TOTAL:		

DINNER			SNACK		
TIME:			TIME:		
LOCATION:			LOCATION:		
FOOD ITEM	CALORIES	CARBS	FOOD ITEM	CALORIES	CARBS
TOTAL:			TOTAL:		

Exercise Activity: Hours ‖ Minutes ‖ Calories Burned

_____

Measurements: Weight ‖ Chest ‖ Waist ‖ Hips

_____

How Do I Feel About
My Progress Today?

BREAKFAST			LUNCH		
TIME:			TIME:		
LOCATION:			LOCATION:		
FOOD ITEM	CALORIES	CARBS	FOOD ITEM	CALORIES	CARBS
TOTAL:			TOTAL:		

DINNER			SNACK		
TIME:			TIME:		
LOCATION:			LOCATION:		
FOOD ITEM	CALORIES	CARBS	FOOD ITEM	CALORIES	CARBS
TOTAL:			TOTAL:		

DATE _____

Exercise Activity: Hours || Minutes || Calories Burned

Measurements: Weight || Chest || Waist || Hips

How Do I Feel About
My Progress Today?

BREAKFAST			LUNCH		
TIME:			TIME:		
LOCATION:			LOCATION:		
FOOD ITEM	CALORIES	CARBS	FOOD ITEM	CALORIES	CARBS
TOTAL:			TOTAL:		

DINNER			SNACK		
TIME:			TIME:		
LOCATION:			LOCATION:		
FOOD ITEM	CALORIES	CARBS	FOOD ITEM	CALORIES	CARBS
TOTAL:			TOTAL:		

Exercise Activity: Hours ‖ Minutes ‖ Calories Burned

Measurements: Weight ‖ Chest ‖ Waist ‖ Hips

How Do I Feel About My Progress Today?

BREAKFAST		
TIME:		
LOCATION:		
FOOD ITEM	CALORIES	CARBS
TOTAL:		

LUNCH		
TIME:		
LOCATION:		
FOOD ITEM	CALORIES	CARBS
TOTAL:		

DINNER		
TIME:		
LOCATION:		
FOOD ITEM	CALORIES	CARBS
TOTAL:		

SNACK		
TIME:		
LOCATION:		
FOOD ITEM	CALORIES	CARBS
TOTAL:		

DATE _____

Exercise Activity: Hours || Minutes || Calories Burned

Measurements: Weight || Chest || Waist || Hips

How Do I Feel About My Progress Today?

BREAKFAST			LUNCH		
TIME:			TIME:		
LOCATION:			LOCATION:		
FOOD ITEM	CALORIES	CARBS	FOOD ITEM	CALORIES	CARBS
TOTAL:			TOTAL:		

DINNER			SNACK		
TIME:			TIME:		
LOCATION:			LOCATION:		
FOOD ITEM	CALORIES	CARBS	FOOD ITEM	CALORIES	CARBS
TOTAL:			TOTAL:		

DATE _____

Exercise Activity: Hours || Minutes || Calories Burned

Measurements: Weight || Chest || Waist || Hips

How Do I Feel About
My Progress Today?

BREAKFAST			LUNCH		
TIME:			TIME:		
LOCATION:			LOCATION:		
FOOD ITEM	CALORIES	CARBS	FOOD ITEM	CALORIES	CARBS
TOTAL:			TOTAL:		

DINNER			SNACK		
TIME:			TIME:		
LOCATION:			LOCATION:		
FOOD ITEM	CALORIES	CARBS	FOOD ITEM	CALORIES	CARBS
TOTAL:			TOTAL:		

DATE _____

Exercise Activity: Hours || Minutes || Calories Burned

Measurements: Weight || Chest || Waist || Hips

How Do I Feel About
My Progress Today?

BREAKFAST			LUNCH		
TIME:			TIME:		
LOCATION:			LOCATION:		
FOOD ITEM	CALORIES	CARBS	FOOD ITEM	CALORIES	CARBS
TOTAL:			TOTAL:		

DINNER			SNACK		
TIME:			TIME:		
LOCATION:			LOCATION:		
FOOD ITEM	CALORIES	CARBS	FOOD ITEM	CALORIES	CARBS
TOTAL:			TOTAL:		

DATE _____

Exercise Activity: Hours || Minutes || Calories Burned

_____

Measurements: Weight || Chest || Waist || Hips

_____

How Do I Feel About
My Progress Today?

BREAKFAST			LUNCH		
TIME:			TIME:		
LOCATION:			LOCATION:		
FOOD ITEM	CALORIES	CARBS	FOOD ITEM	CALORIES	CARBS
TOTAL:			TOTAL:		

DINNER			SNACK		
TIME:			TIME:		
LOCATION:			LOCATION:		
FOOD ITEM	CALORIES	CARBS	FOOD ITEM	CALORIES	CARBS
TOTAL:			TOTAL:		

DATE _____

Exercise Activity: Hours || Minutes || Calories Burned

Measurements: Weight || Chest || Waist || Hips

How Do I Feel About
My Progress Today?

BREAKFAST			LUNCH		
TIME:			TIME:		
LOCATION:			LOCATION:		
FOOD ITEM	CALORIES	CARBS	FOOD ITEM	CALORIES	CARBS
TOTAL:			TOTAL:		

DINNER			SNACK		
TIME:			TIME:		
LOCATION:			LOCATION:		
FOOD ITEM	CALORIES	CARBS	FOOD ITEM	CALORIES	CARBS
TOTAL:			TOTAL:		

DATE _____

Exercise Activity: Hours || Minutes || Calories Burned

_____

Measurements: Weight || Chest || Waist || Hips

_____

How Do I Feel About
My Progress Today?

BREAKFAST			LUNCH		
TIME:			TIME:		
LOCATION:			LOCATION:		
FOOD ITEM	CALORIES	CARBS	FOOD ITEM	CALORIES	CARBS
TOTAL:			TOTAL:		

DINNER			SNACK		
TIME:			TIME:		
LOCATION:			LOCATION:		
FOOD ITEM	CALORIES	CARBS	FOOD ITEM	CALORIES	CARBS
TOTAL:			TOTAL:		

DATE _____

Exercise Activity: Hours || Minutes || Calories Burned

Measurements: Weight || Chest || Waist || Hips

How Do I Feel About My Progress Today?

BREAKFAST				LUNCH		
TIME:				TIME:		
LOCATION:				LOCATION:		
FOOD ITEM		CALORIES	CARBS	FOOD ITEM		CALORIES	CARBS
TOTAL:				TOTAL:		

DINNER				SNACK		
TIME:				TIME:		
LOCATION:				LOCATION:		
FOOD ITEM		CALORIES	CARBS	FOOD ITEM		CALORIES	CARBS
TOTAL:				TOTAL:		

Exercise Activity: Hours || Minutes || Calories Burned

Measurements: Weight || Chest || Waist || Hips

How Do I Feel About
My Progress Today?

BREAKFAST			LUNCH		
TIME:			TIME:		
LOCATION:			LOCATION:		
FOOD ITEM	CALORIES	CARBS	FOOD ITEM	CALORIES	CARBS
TOTAL:			TOTAL:		

DINNER			SNACK		
TIME:			TIME:		
LOCATION:			LOCATION:		
FOOD ITEM	CALORIES	CARBS	FOOD ITEM	CALORIES	CARBS
TOTAL:			TOTAL:		

Exercise Activity: Hours || Minutes || Calories Burned

Measurements: Weight || Chest || Waist || Hips

How Do I Feel About My Progress Today?

BREAKFAST			**LUNCH**		
TIME:			TIME:		
LOCATION:			LOCATION:		
FOOD ITEM	CALORIES	CARBS	FOOD ITEM	CALORIES	CARBS
TOTAL:			TOTAL:		

DINNER			**SNACK**		
TIME:			TIME:		
LOCATION:			LOCATION:		
FOOD ITEM	CALORIES	CARBS	FOOD ITEM	CALORIES	CARBS
TOTAL:			TOTAL:		

DATE _____

Exercise Activity: Hours ‖ Minutes ‖ Calories Burned

Measurements: Weight ‖ Chest ‖ Waist ‖ Hips

How Do I Feel About
My Progress Today?

BREAKFAST			LUNCH		
TIME:			TIME:		
LOCATION:			LOCATION:		
FOOD ITEM	CALORIES	CARBS	FOOD ITEM	CALORIES	CARBS
TOTAL:			TOTAL:		

DINNER			SNACK		
TIME:			TIME:		
LOCATION:			LOCATION:		
FOOD ITEM	CALORIES	CARBS	FOOD ITEM	CALORIES	CARBS
TOTAL:			TOTAL:		

DATE _____

Exercise Activity: Hours || Minutes || Calories Burned

Measurements: Weight || Chest || Waist || Hips

How Do I Feel About
My Progress Today?

BREAKFAST			LUNCH		
TIME:			TIME:		
LOCATION:			LOCATION:		
FOOD ITEM	CALORIES	CARBS	FOOD ITEM	CALORIES	CARBS
TOTAL:			TOTAL:		

DINNER			SNACK		
TIME:			TIME:		
LOCATION:			LOCATION:		
FOOD ITEM	CALORIES	CARBS	FOOD ITEM	CALORIES	CARBS
TOTAL:			TOTAL:		

DATE _____

Exercise Activity: Hours || Minutes || Calories Burned

_____

Measurements: Weight || Chest || Waist || Hips

_____

How Do I Feel About My Progress Today?

BREAKFAST			LUNCH		
TIME:			TIME:		
LOCATION:			LOCATION:		
FOOD ITEM	CALORIES	CARBS	FOOD ITEM	CALORIES	CARBS
TOTAL:			TOTAL:		

DINNER			SNACK		
TIME:			TIME:		
LOCATION:			LOCATION:		
FOOD ITEM	CALORIES	CARBS	FOOD ITEM	CALORIES	CARBS
TOTAL:			TOTAL:		

Exercise Activity: Hours || Minutes || Calories Burned

Measurements: Weight || Chest || Waist || Hips

How Do I Feel About
My Progress Today?

BREAKFAST		
TIME:		
LOCATION:		
FOOD ITEM	CALORIES	CARBS
TOTAL:		

LUNCH		
TIME:		
LOCATION:		
FOOD ITEM	CALORIES	CARBS
TOTAL:		

DINNER		
TIME:		
LOCATION:		
FOOD ITEM	CALORIES	CARBS
TOTAL:		

SNACK		
TIME:		
LOCATION:		
FOOD ITEM	CALORIES	CARBS
TOTAL:		

DATE _____

Exercise Activity: Hours ‖ Minutes ‖ Calories Burned

Measurements: Weight ‖ Chest ‖ Waist ‖ Hips

How Do I Feel About
My Progress Today?

BREAKFAST			LUNCH		
TIME:			TIME:		
LOCATION:			LOCATION:		
FOOD ITEM	CALORIES	CARBS	FOOD ITEM	CALORIES	CARBS
TOTAL:			TOTAL:		

DINNER			SNACK		
TIME:			TIME:		
LOCATION:			LOCATION:		
FOOD ITEM	CALORIES	CARBS	FOOD ITEM	CALORIES	CARBS
TOTAL:			TOTAL:		

DATE _____

Exercise Activity: Hours ‖ Minutes ‖ Calories Burned

Measurements: Weight ‖ Chest ‖ Waist ‖ Hips

How Do I Feel About
My Progress Today?

BREAKFAST			LUNCH		
TIME:			TIME:		
LOCATION:			LOCATION:		
FOOD ITEM	CALORIES	CARBS	FOOD ITEM	CALORIES	CARBS
TOTAL:			TOTAL:		

DINNER			SNACK		
TIME:			TIME:		
LOCATION:			LOCATION:		
FOOD ITEM	CALORIES	CARBS	FOOD ITEM	CALORIES	CARBS
TOTAL:			TOTAL:		

DATE _____

Exercise Activity: Hours ‖ Minutes ‖ Calories Burned

Measurements: Weight ‖ Chest ‖ Waist ‖ Hips

How Do I Feel About
My Progress Today?

BREAKFAST			LUNCH		
TIME:			TIME:		
LOCATION:			LOCATION:		
FOOD ITEM	CALORIES	CARBS	FOOD ITEM	CALORIES	CARBS
TOTAL:			TOTAL:		

DINNER			SNACK		
TIME:			TIME:		
LOCATION:			LOCATION:		
FOOD ITEM	CALORIES	CARBS	FOOD ITEM	CALORIES	CARBS
TOTAL:			TOTAL:		

Exercise Activity:　Hours　||　Minutes　||　Calories Burned

Measurements: Weight　||　Chest　||　Waist　||　Hips

How Do I Feel About
My Progress Today?

BREAKFAST			LUNCH		
TIME:			TIME:		
LOCATION:			LOCATION:		
FOOD ITEM	CALORIES	CARBS	FOOD ITEM	CALORIES	CARBS
TOTAL:			TOTAL:		

DINNER			SNACK		
TIME:			TIME:		
LOCATION:			LOCATION:		
FOOD ITEM	CALORIES	CARBS	FOOD ITEM	CALORIES	CARBS
TOTAL:			TOTAL:		

DATE _____

Exercise Activity:　Hours　||　Minutes　||　Calories Burned

Measurements: Weight　||　Chest　||　Waist　||　Hips

How Do I Feel About
My Progress Today?

BREAKFAST				LUNCH		
TIME:				TIME:		
LOCATION:				LOCATION:		
FOOD ITEM		CALORIES	CARBS	FOOD ITEM		CALORIES	CARBS
TOTAL:				TOTAL:		

DINNER				SNACK		
TIME:				TIME:		
LOCATION:				LOCATION:		
FOOD ITEM		CALORIES	CARBS	FOOD ITEM		CALORIES	CARBS
TOTAL:				TOTAL:		

Exercise Activity: Hours || Minutes || Calories Burned

Measurements: Weight || Chest || Waist || Hips

How Do I Feel About
My Progress Today?

BREAKFAST			LUNCH		
TIME:			TIME:		
LOCATION:			LOCATION:		
FOOD ITEM	CALORIES	CARBS	FOOD ITEM	CALORIES	CARBS
TOTAL:			TOTAL:		
DINNER			SNACK		
TIME:			TIME:		
LOCATION:			LOCATION:		
FOOD ITEM	CALORIES	CARBS	FOOD ITEM	CALORIES	CARBS
TOTAL:			TOTAL:		

DATE _____

Exercise Activity: Hours || Minutes || Calories Burned

Measurements: Weight || Chest || Waist || Hips

How Do I Feel About
My Progress Today?   😄   😌   😛   😟   😫

BREAKFAST				LUNCH		
TIME:				TIME:		
LOCATION:				LOCATION:		
FOOD ITEM		CALORIES	CARBS	FOOD ITEM		CALORIES	CARBS
TOTAL:				TOTAL:		

DINNER				SNACK		
TIME:				TIME:		
LOCATION:				LOCATION:		
FOOD ITEM		CALORIES	CARBS	FOOD ITEM		CALORIES	CARBS
TOTAL:				TOTAL:		

DATE _____

Exercise Activity: Hours ‖ Minutes ‖ Calories Burned

_____

Measurements: Weight ‖ Chest ‖ Waist ‖ Hips

_____

How Do I Feel About
My Progress Today?

BREAKFAST			LUNCH		
TIME:			TIME:		
LOCATION:			LOCATION:		
FOOD ITEM	CALORIES	CARBS	FOOD ITEM	CALORIES	CARBS
TOTAL:			TOTAL:		

DINNER			SNACK		
TIME:			TIME:		
LOCATION:			LOCATION:		
FOOD ITEM	CALORIES	CARBS	FOOD ITEM	CALORIES	CARBS
TOTAL:			TOTAL:		

DATE _____

Exercise Activity: Hours || Minutes || Calories Burned

_____

Measurements: Weight || Chest || Waist || Hips

_____

How Do I Feel About
My Progress Today?

BREAKFAST			LUNCH		
TIME:			TIME:		
LOCATION:			LOCATION:		
FOOD ITEM	CALORIES	CARBS	FOOD ITEM	CALORIES	CARBS
TOTAL:			TOTAL:		

DINNER			SNACK		
TIME:			TIME:		
LOCATION:			LOCATION:		
FOOD ITEM	CALORIES	CARBS	FOOD ITEM	CALORIES	CARBS
TOTAL:			TOTAL:		

DATE _____

Exercise Activity: Hours || Minutes || Calories Burned

_____

Measurements: Weight || Chest || Waist || Hips

_____

How Do I Feel About
My Progress Today?

BREAKFAST			LUNCH		
TIME:			TIME:		
LOCATION:			LOCATION:		
FOOD ITEM	CALORIES	CARBS	FOOD ITEM	CALORIES	CARBS
TOTAL:			TOTAL:		

DINNER			SNACK		
TIME:			TIME:		
LOCATION:			LOCATION:		
FOOD ITEM	CALORIES	CARBS	FOOD ITEM	CALORIES	CARBS
TOTAL:			TOTAL:		

DATE _____

Exercise Activity: Hours || Minutes || Calories Burned

_____

Measurements: Weight || Chest || Waist || Hips

_____

How Do I Feel About
My Progress Today?

BREAKFAST			LUNCH		
TIME:			TIME:		
LOCATION:			LOCATION:		
FOOD ITEM	CALORIES	CARBS	FOOD ITEM	CALORIES	CARBS
TOTAL:			TOTAL:		

DINNER			SNACK		
TIME:			TIME:		
LOCATION:			LOCATION:		
FOOD ITEM	CALORIES	CARBS	FOOD ITEM	CALORIES	CARBS
TOTAL:			TOTAL:		

DATE _____

Exercise Activity: Hours || Minutes || Calories Burned

Measurements: Weight || Chest || Waist || Hips

How Do I Feel About
My Progress Today?

BREAKFAST			LUNCH		
TIME:			TIME:		
LOCATION:			LOCATION:		
FOOD ITEM	CALORIES	CARBS	FOOD ITEM	CALORIES	CARBS
TOTAL:			TOTAL:		

DINNER			SNACK		
TIME:			TIME:		
LOCATION:			LOCATION:		
FOOD ITEM	CALORIES	CARBS	FOOD ITEM	CALORIES	CARBS
TOTAL:			TOTAL:		

DATE _____

Exercise Activity: Hours || Minutes || Calories Burned

_____

Measurements: Weight || Chest || Waist || Hips

_____

How Do I Feel About
My Progress Today?

BREAKFAST			LUNCH		
TIME:			TIME:		
LOCATION:			LOCATION:		
FOOD ITEM	CALORIES	CARBS	FOOD ITEM	CALORIES	CARBS
TOTAL:			TOTAL:		

DINNER			SNACK		
TIME:			TIME:		
LOCATION:			LOCATION:		
FOOD ITEM	CALORIES	CARBS	FOOD ITEM	CALORIES	CARBS
TOTAL:			TOTAL:		

DATE _____

Exercise Activity: Hours ‖ Minutes ‖ Calories Burned

Measurements: Weight ‖ Chest ‖ Waist ‖ Hips

How Do I Feel About
My Progress Today?

BREAKFAST			LUNCH		
TIME:			TIME:		
LOCATION:			LOCATION:		
FOOD ITEM	CALORIES	CARBS	FOOD ITEM	CALORIES	CARBS
TOTAL:			TOTAL:		

DINNER			SNACK		
TIME:			TIME:		
LOCATION:			LOCATION:		
FOOD ITEM	CALORIES	CARBS	FOOD ITEM	CALORIES	CARBS
TOTAL:			TOTAL:		

DATE _____

Exercise Activity: Hours || Minutes || Calories Burned

Measurements: Weight || Chest || Waist || Hips

How Do I Feel About
My Progress Today?

BREAKFAST			LUNCH		
TIME:			TIME:		
LOCATION:			LOCATION:		
FOOD ITEM	CALORIES	CARBS	FOOD ITEM	CALORIES	CARBS
TOTAL:			TOTAL:		

DINNER			SNACK		
TIME:			TIME:		
LOCATION:			LOCATION:		
FOOD ITEM	CALORIES	CARBS	FOOD ITEM	CALORIES	CARBS
TOTAL:			TOTAL:		

Exercise Activity: Hours || Minutes || Calories Burned

Measurements: Weight || Chest || Waist || Hips

How Do I Feel About
My Progress Today?

BREAKFAST			**LUNCH**		
TIME:			TIME:		
LOCATION:			LOCATION:		
FOOD ITEM	| CALORIES	| CARBS	FOOD ITEM	| CALORIES	| CARBS
TOTAL:			TOTAL:		
DINNER			**SNACK**		
TIME:			TIME:		
LOCATION:			LOCATION:		
FOOD ITEM	| CALORIES	| CARBS	FOOD ITEM	| CALORIES	| CARBS
TOTAL:			TOTAL:		

DATE _____

Exercise Activity: Hours || Minutes || Calories Burned

Measurements: Weight || Chest || Waist || Hips

How Do I Feel About
My Progress Today?

BREAKFAST			LUNCH		
TIME:			TIME:		
LOCATION:			LOCATION:		
FOOD ITEM	CALORIES	CARBS	FOOD ITEM	CALORIES	CARBS
TOTAL:			TOTAL:		

DINNER			SNACK		
TIME:			TIME:		
LOCATION:			LOCATION:		
FOOD ITEM	CALORIES	CARBS	FOOD ITEM	CALORIES	CARBS
TOTAL:			TOTAL:		

DATE _____

Exercise Activity: Hours ‖ Minutes ‖ Calories Burned

Measurements: Weight ‖ Chest ‖ Waist ‖ Hips

How Do I Feel About
My Progress Today?

BREAKFAST		
TIME:		
LOCATION:		
FOOD ITEM	CALORIES	CARBS
TOTAL:		

LUNCH		
TIME:		
LOCATION:		
FOOD ITEM	CALORIES	CARBS
TOTAL:		

DINNER		
TIME:		
LOCATION:		
FOOD ITEM	CALORIES	CARBS
TOTAL:		

SNACK		
TIME:		
LOCATION:		
FOOD ITEM	CALORIES	CARBS
TOTAL:		

Exercise Activity: Hours || Minutes || Calories Burned

Measurements: Weight || Chest || Waist || Hips

How Do I Feel About
My Progress Today?

BREAKFAST			LUNCH		
TIME:			TIME:		
LOCATION:			LOCATION:		
FOOD ITEM	CALORIES	CARBS	FOOD ITEM	CALORIES	CARBS
TOTAL:			TOTAL:		

DINNER			SNACK		
TIME:			TIME:		
LOCATION:			LOCATION:		
FOOD ITEM	CALORIES	CARBS	FOOD ITEM	CALORIES	CARBS
TOTAL:			TOTAL:		

DATE _____

Exercise Activity: Hours || Minutes || Calories Burned

Measurements: Weight || Chest || Waist || Hips

How Do I Feel About
My Progress Today?

BREAKFAST			LUNCH		
TIME:			TIME:		
LOCATION:			LOCATION:		
FOOD ITEM	CALORIES	CARBS	FOOD ITEM	CALORIES	CARBS
TOTAL:			TOTAL:		

DINNER			SNACK		
TIME:			TIME:		
LOCATION:			LOCATION:		
FOOD ITEM	CALORIES	CARBS	FOOD ITEM	CALORIES	CARBS
TOTAL:			TOTAL:		

DATE _____

Exercise Activity: Hours || Minutes || Calories Burned

_____

Measurements: Weight || Chest || Waist || Hips

_____

How Do I Feel About
My Progress Today?

BREAKFAST			LUNCH		
TIME:			TIME:		
LOCATION:			LOCATION:		
FOOD ITEM	CALORIES	CARBS	FOOD ITEM	CALORIES	CARBS
TOTAL:			TOTAL:		

DINNER			SNACK		
TIME:			TIME:		
LOCATION:			LOCATION:		
FOOD ITEM	CALORIES	CARBS	FOOD ITEM	CALORIES	CARBS
TOTAL:			TOTAL:		

DATE _____

Exercise Activity: Hours || Minutes || Calories Burned

Measurements: Weight || Chest || Waist || Hips

How Do I Feel About
My Progress Today?

BREAKFAST			LUNCH		
TIME:			TIME:		
LOCATION:			LOCATION:		
FOOD ITEM	CALORIES	CARBS	FOOD ITEM	CALORIES	CARBS
TOTAL:			TOTAL:		

DINNER			SNACK		
TIME:			TIME:		
LOCATION:			LOCATION:		
FOOD ITEM	CALORIES	CARBS	FOOD ITEM	CALORIES	CARBS
TOTAL:			TOTAL:		

DATE _____

Exercise Activity: Hours || Minutes || Calories Burned

Measurements: Weight || Chest || Waist || Hips

How Do I Feel About My Progress Today?

BREAKFAST			LUNCH		
TIME:			TIME:		
LOCATION:			LOCATION:		
FOOD ITEM	CALORIES	CARBS	FOOD ITEM	CALORIES	CARBS
TOTAL:			TOTAL:		

DINNER			SNACK		
TIME:			TIME:		
LOCATION:			LOCATION:		
FOOD ITEM	CALORIES	CARBS	FOOD ITEM	CALORIES	CARBS
TOTAL:			TOTAL:		

DATE _____

Exercise Activity: Hours || Minutes || Calories Burned

Measurements: Weight || Chest || Waist || Hips

How Do I Feel About
My Progress Today?

BREAKFAST			LUNCH		
TIME:			TIME:		
LOCATION:			LOCATION:		
FOOD ITEM	CALORIES	CARBS	FOOD ITEM	CALORIES	CARBS
TOTAL:			TOTAL:		

DINNER			SNACK		
TIME:			TIME:		
LOCATION:			LOCATION:		
FOOD ITEM	CALORIES	CARBS	FOOD ITEM	CALORIES	CARBS
TOTAL:			TOTAL:		

DATE _____

Exercise Activity: Hours || Minutes || Calories Burned

_____

Measurements: Weight || Chest || Waist || Hips

_____

How Do I Feel About
My Progress Today?

BREAKFAST		
TIME:		
LOCATION:		
FOOD ITEM	CALORIES	CARBS
TOTAL:		

LUNCH		
TIME:		
LOCATION:		
FOOD ITEM	CALORIES	CARBS
TOTAL:		

DINNER		
TIME:		
LOCATION:		
FOOD ITEM	CALORIES	CARBS
TOTAL:		

SNACK		
TIME:		
LOCATION:		
FOOD ITEM	CALORIES	CARBS
TOTAL:		

DATE _____

Exercise Activity: Hours || Minutes || Calories Burned

Measurements: Weight || Chest || Waist || Hips

How Do I Feel About
My Progress Today?

BREAKFAST			LUNCH		
TIME:			TIME:		
LOCATION:			LOCATION:		
FOOD ITEM	CALORIES	CARBS	FOOD ITEM	CALORIES	CARBS
TOTAL:			TOTAL:		

DINNER			SNACK		
TIME:			TIME:		
LOCATION:			LOCATION:		
FOOD ITEM	CALORIES	CARBS	FOOD ITEM	CALORIES	CARBS
TOTAL:			TOTAL:		

DATE _____

Exercise Activity: Hours ‖ Minutes ‖ Calories Burned

Measurements: Weight ‖ Chest ‖ Waist ‖ Hips

How Do I Feel About My Progress Today?

BREAKFAST			LUNCH		
TIME:			TIME:		
LOCATION:			LOCATION:		
FOOD ITEM	CALORIES	CARBS	FOOD ITEM	CALORIES	CARBS
TOTAL:			TOTAL:		

DINNER			SNACK		
TIME:			TIME:		
LOCATION:			LOCATION:		
FOOD ITEM	CALORIES	CARBS	FOOD ITEM	CALORIES	CARBS
TOTAL:			TOTAL:		

DATE _____

Exercise Activity: Hours || Minutes || Calories Burned

Measurements: Weight || Chest || Waist || Hips

How Do I Feel About My Progress Today?

BREAKFAST			LUNCH		
TIME:			TIME:		
LOCATION:			LOCATION:		
FOOD ITEM	CALORIES	CARBS	FOOD ITEM	CALORIES	CARBS
TOTAL:			TOTAL:		

DINNER			SNACK		
TIME:			TIME:		
LOCATION:			LOCATION:		
FOOD ITEM	CALORIES	CARBS	FOOD ITEM	CALORIES	CARBS
TOTAL:			TOTAL:		

DATE _____

Exercise Activity: Hours || Minutes || Calories Burned

Measurements: Weight || Chest || Waist || Hips

How Do I Feel About
My Progress Today?

BREAKFAST			LUNCH		
TIME:			TIME:		
LOCATION:			LOCATION:		
FOOD ITEM	CALORIES	CARBS	FOOD ITEM	CALORIES	CARBS
TOTAL:			TOTAL:		

DINNER			SNACK		
TIME:			TIME:		
LOCATION:			LOCATION:		
FOOD ITEM	CALORIES	CARBS	FOOD ITEM	CALORIES	CARBS
TOTAL:			TOTAL:		

Exercise Activity: Hours || Minutes || Calories Burned

Measurements: Weight || Chest || Waist || Hips

How Do I Feel About
My Progress Today?

BREAKFAST			LUNCH		
TIME:			TIME:		
LOCATION:			LOCATION:		
FOOD ITEM	CALORIES	CARBS	FOOD ITEM	CALORIES	CARBS
TOTAL:			TOTAL:		

DINNER			SNACK		
TIME:			TIME:		
LOCATION:			LOCATION:		
FOOD ITEM	CALORIES	CARBS	FOOD ITEM	CALORIES	CARBS
TOTAL:			TOTAL:		

Exercise Activity: Hours ‖ Minutes ‖ Calories Burned

Measurements: Weight ‖ Chest ‖ Waist ‖ Hips

How Do I Feel About
My Progress Today?

BREAKFAST				LUNCH		
TIME:				TIME:		
LOCATION:				LOCATION:		
FOOD ITEM	CALORIES	CARBS		FOOD ITEM	CALORIES	CARBS
TOTAL:				TOTAL:		

DINNER				SNACK		
TIME:				TIME:		
LOCATION:				LOCATION:		
FOOD ITEM	CALORIES	CARBS		FOOD ITEM	CALORIES	CARBS
TOTAL:				TOTAL:		

DATE _____

Exercise Activity: Hours || Minutes || Calories Burned

Measurements: Weight || Chest || Waist || Hips

How Do I Feel About
My Progress Today?

BREAKFAST			LUNCH		
TIME:			TIME:		
LOCATION:			LOCATION:		
FOOD ITEM	CALORIES	CARBS	FOOD ITEM	CALORIES	CARBS
TOTAL:			TOTAL:		

DINNER			SNACK		
TIME:			TIME:		
LOCATION:			LOCATION:		
FOOD ITEM	CALORIES	CARBS	FOOD ITEM	CALORIES	CARBS
TOTAL:			TOTAL:		

DATE _____

Exercise Activity: Hours ‖ Minutes ‖ Calories Burned

_____

Measurements: Weight ‖ Chest ‖ Waist ‖ Hips

_____

How Do I Feel About
My Progress Today?

BREAKFAST			LUNCH		
TIME:			TIME:		
LOCATION:			LOCATION:		
FOOD ITEM	CALORIES	CARBS	FOOD ITEM	CALORIES	CARBS
TOTAL:			TOTAL:		

DINNER			SNACK		
TIME:			TIME:		
LOCATION:			LOCATION:		
FOOD ITEM	CALORIES	CARBS	FOOD ITEM	CALORIES	CARBS
TOTAL:			TOTAL:		

Exercise Activity: Hours || Minutes || Calories Burned

Measurements: Weight || Chest || Waist || Hips

How Do I Feel About
My Progress Today?

BREAKFAST			LUNCH		
TIME:			TIME:		
LOCATION:			LOCATION:		
FOOD ITEM	CALORIES	CARBS	FOOD ITEM	CALORIES	CARBS
TOTAL:			TOTAL:		

DINNER			SNACK		
TIME:			TIME:		
LOCATION:			LOCATION:		
FOOD ITEM	CALORIES	CARBS	FOOD ITEM	CALORIES	CARBS
TOTAL:			TOTAL:		

DATE _____

Exercise Activity: Hours || Minutes || Calories Burned

Measurements: Weight || Chest || Waist || Hips

How Do I Feel About
My Progress Today?

BREAKFAST			LUNCH		
TIME:			TIME:		
LOCATION:			LOCATION:		
FOOD ITEM	CALORIES	CARBS	FOOD ITEM	CALORIES	CARBS
TOTAL:			TOTAL:		

DINNER			SNACK		
TIME:			TIME:		
LOCATION:			LOCATION:		
FOOD ITEM	CALORIES	CARBS	FOOD ITEM	CALORIES	CARBS
TOTAL:			TOTAL:		

Exercise Activity: Hours ‖ Minutes ‖ Calories Burned

Measurements: Weight ‖ Chest ‖ Waist ‖ Hips

How Do I Feel About
My Progress Today?

BREAKFAST			LUNCH		
TIME:			TIME:		
LOCATION:			LOCATION:		
FOOD ITEM	CALORIES	CARBS	FOOD ITEM	CALORIES	CARBS
TOTAL:			TOTAL:		

DINNER			SNACK		
TIME:			TIME:		
LOCATION:			LOCATION:		
FOOD ITEM	CALORIES	CARBS	FOOD ITEM	CALORIES	CARBS
TOTAL:			TOTAL:		

DATE _____

Exercise Activity: Hours || Minutes || Calories Burned

Measurements: Weight || Chest || Waist || Hips

How Do I Feel About
My Progress Today?

BREAKFAST			LUNCH		
TIME:			TIME:		
LOCATION:			LOCATION:		
FOOD ITEM	CALORIES	CARBS	FOOD ITEM	CALORIES	CARBS
TOTAL:			TOTAL:		
DINNER			**SNACK**		
TIME:			TIME:		
LOCATION:			LOCATION:		
FOOD ITEM	CALORIES	CARBS	FOOD ITEM	CALORIES	CARBS
TOTAL:			TOTAL:		

Exercise Activity: Hours || Minutes || Calories Burned

Measurements: Weight || Chest || Waist || Hips

How Do I Feel About
My Progress Today?

BREAKFAST			LUNCH		
TIME:			TIME:		
LOCATION:			LOCATION:		
FOOD ITEM	CALORIES	CARBS	FOOD ITEM	CALORIES	CARBS
TOTAL:			TOTAL:		

DINNER			SNACK		
TIME:			TIME:		
LOCATION:			LOCATION:		
FOOD ITEM	CALORIES	CARBS	FOOD ITEM	CALORIES	CARBS
TOTAL:			TOTAL:		

DATE _____

Exercise Activity: Hours || Minutes || Calories Burned

Measurements: Weight || Chest || Waist || Hips

How Do I Feel About
My Progress Today?

BREAKFAST			LUNCH		
TIME:			TIME:		
LOCATION:			LOCATION:		
FOOD ITEM	CALORIES	CARBS	FOOD ITEM	CALORIES	CARBS
TOTAL:			TOTAL:		

DINNER			SNACK		
TIME:			TIME:		
LOCATION:			LOCATION:		
FOOD ITEM	CALORIES	CARBS	FOOD ITEM	CALORIES	CARBS
TOTAL:			TOTAL:		

Exercise Activity: Hours || Minutes || Calories Burned

_____

Measurements: Weight || Chest || Waist || Hips

_____

How Do I Feel About
My Progress Today?

BREAKFAST			LUNCH		
TIME:			TIME:		
LOCATION:			LOCATION:		
FOOD ITEM	CALORIES	CARBS	FOOD ITEM	CALORIES	CARBS
TOTAL:			TOTAL:		
DINNER			SNACK		
TIME:			TIME:		
LOCATION:			LOCATION:		
FOOD ITEM	CALORIES	CARBS	FOOD ITEM	CALORIES	CARBS
TOTAL:			TOTAL:		

Exercise Activity: Hours || Minutes || Calories Burned

_____

Measurements: Weight || Chest || Waist || Hips

_____

How Do I Feel About
My Progress Today?

BREAKFAST			LUNCH		
TIME:			TIME:		
LOCATION:			LOCATION:		
FOOD ITEM	CALORIES	CARBS	FOOD ITEM	CALORIES	CARBS
TOTAL:			TOTAL:		

DINNER			SNACK		
TIME:			TIME:		
LOCATION:			LOCATION:		
FOOD ITEM	CALORIES	CARBS	FOOD ITEM	CALORIES	CARBS
TOTAL:			TOTAL:		

DATE _____

Exercise Activity: Hours || Minutes || Calories Burned

Measurements: Weight || Chest || Waist || Hips

How Do I Feel About
My Progress Today?

BREAKFAST			LUNCH		
TIME:			TIME:		
LOCATION:			LOCATION:		
FOOD ITEM	CALORIES	CARBS	FOOD ITEM	CALORIES	CARBS
TOTAL:			TOTAL:		

DINNER			SNACK		
TIME:			TIME:		
LOCATION:			LOCATION:		
FOOD ITEM	CALORIES	CARBS	FOOD ITEM	CALORIES	CARBS
TOTAL:			TOTAL:		

DATE _____

Exercise Activity: Hours || Minutes || Calories Burned

Measurements: Weight || Chest || Waist || Hips

How Do I Feel About My Progress Today?

BREAKFAST			LUNCH		
TIME:			TIME:		
LOCATION:			LOCATION:		
FOOD ITEM	CALORIES	CARBS	FOOD ITEM	CALORIES	CARBS
TOTAL:			TOTAL:		

DINNER			SNACK		
TIME:			TIME:		
LOCATION:			LOCATION:		
FOOD ITEM	CALORIES	CARBS	FOOD ITEM	CALORIES	CARBS
TOTAL:			TOTAL:		

DATE _____

Exercise Activity: Hours || Minutes || Calories Burned

Measurements: Weight || Chest || Waist || Hips

How Do I Feel About
My Progress Today?

BREAKFAST			LUNCH		
TIME:			TIME:		
LOCATION:			LOCATION:		
FOOD ITEM	CALORIES	CARBS	FOOD ITEM	CALORIES	CARBS
TOTAL:			TOTAL:		

DINNER			SNACK		
TIME:			TIME:		
LOCATION:			LOCATION:		
FOOD ITEM	CALORIES	CARBS	FOOD ITEM	CALORIES	CARBS
TOTAL:			TOTAL:		

Exercise Activity: Hours || Minutes || Calories Burned

Measurements: Weight || Chest || Waist || Hips

How Do I Feel About
My Progress Today?

BREAKFAST			LUNCH		
TIME:			TIME:		
LOCATION:			LOCATION:		
FOOD ITEM	CALORIES	CARBS	FOOD ITEM	CALORIES	CARBS
TOTAL:			TOTAL:		

DINNER			SNACK		
TIME:			TIME:		
LOCATION:			LOCATION:		
FOOD ITEM	CALORIES	CARBS	FOOD ITEM	CALORIES	CARBS
TOTAL:			TOTAL:		

DATE _____

Exercise Activity: Hours ‖ Minutes ‖ Calories Burned

Measurements: Weight ‖ Chest ‖ Waist ‖ Hips

How Do I Feel About
My Progress Today?

BREAKFAST			LUNCH		
TIME:			TIME:		
LOCATION:			LOCATION:		
FOOD ITEM	CALORIES	CARBS	FOOD ITEM	CALORIES	CARBS
TOTAL:			TOTAL:		

DINNER			SNACK		
TIME:			TIME:		
LOCATION:			LOCATION:		
FOOD ITEM	CALORIES	CARBS	FOOD ITEM	CALORIES	CARBS
TOTAL:			TOTAL:		

DATE _____

Exercise Activity: Hours ‖ Minutes ‖ Calories Burned

_____

Measurements: Weight ‖ Chest ‖ Waist ‖ Hips

_____

How Do I Feel About
My Progress Today?

BREAKFAST			LUNCH		
TIME:			TIME:		
LOCATION:			LOCATION:		
FOOD ITEM	CALORIES	CARBS	FOOD ITEM	CALORIES	CARBS
TOTAL:			TOTAL:		
DINNER			**SNACK**		
TIME:			TIME:		
LOCATION:			LOCATION:		
FOOD ITEM	CALORIES	CARBS	FOOD ITEM	CALORIES	CARBS
TOTAL:			TOTAL:		

DATE _____

Exercise Activity: Hours || Minutes || Calories Burned

Measurements: Weight || Chest || Waist || Hips

How Do I Feel About
My Progress Today?

BREAKFAST			LUNCH		
TIME:			TIME:		
LOCATION:			LOCATION:		
FOOD ITEM	CALORIES	CARBS	FOOD ITEM	CALORIES	CARBS
TOTAL:			TOTAL:		
DINNER			**SNACK**		
TIME:			TIME:		
LOCATION:			LOCATION:		
FOOD ITEM	CALORIES	CARBS	FOOD ITEM	CALORIES	CARBS
TOTAL:			TOTAL:		

DATE _____

Exercise Activity: Hours || Minutes || Calories Burned

Measurements: Weight || Chest || Waist || Hips

How Do I Feel About
My Progress Today?

BREAKFAST		
TIME:		
LOCATION:		
FOOD ITEM	CALORIES	CARBS
TOTAL:		

LUNCH		
TIME:		
LOCATION:		
FOOD ITEM	CALORIES	CARBS
TOTAL:		

DINNER		
TIME:		
LOCATION:		
FOOD ITEM	CALORIES	CARBS
TOTAL:		

SNACK		
TIME:		
LOCATION:		
FOOD ITEM	CALORIES	CARBS
TOTAL:		

DATE _____

Exercise Activity: Hours || Minutes || Calories Burned

Measurements: Weight || Chest || Waist || Hips

How Do I Feel About My Progress Today?

BREAKFAST			LUNCH		
TIME:			TIME:		
LOCATION:			LOCATION:		
FOOD ITEM	CALORIES	CARBS	FOOD ITEM	CALORIES	CARBS
TOTAL:			TOTAL:		

DINNER			SNACK		
TIME:			TIME:		
LOCATION:			LOCATION:		
FOOD ITEM	CALORIES	CARBS	FOOD ITEM	CALORIES	CARBS
TOTAL:			TOTAL:		

DATE _____

Exercise Activity: Hours ‖ Minutes ‖ Calories Burned

_____

Measurements: Weight ‖ Chest ‖ Waist ‖ Hips

_____

How Do I Feel About
My Progress Today?

BREAKFAST			LUNCH		
TIME:			TIME:		
LOCATION:			LOCATION:		
FOOD ITEM	CALORIES	CARBS	FOOD ITEM	CALORIES	CARBS
TOTAL:			TOTAL:		

DINNER			SNACK		
TIME:			TIME:		
LOCATION:			LOCATION:		
FOOD ITEM	CALORIES	CARBS	FOOD ITEM	CALORIES	CARBS
TOTAL:			TOTAL:		

Exercise Activity: Hours || Minutes || Calories Burned

Measurements: Weight || Chest || Waist || Hips

How Do I Feel About
My Progress Today?

BREAKFAST			**LUNCH**		
TIME:			TIME:		
LOCATION:			LOCATION:		
FOOD ITEM	CALORIES	CARBS	FOOD ITEM	CALORIES	CARBS
TOTAL:			TOTAL:		

DINNER			**SNACK**		
TIME:			TIME:		
LOCATION:			LOCATION:		
FOOD ITEM	CALORIES	CARBS	FOOD ITEM	CALORIES	CARBS
TOTAL:			TOTAL:		

DATE _____

Exercise Activity: Hours ‖ Minutes ‖ Calories Burned

Measurements: Weight ‖ Chest ‖ Waist ‖ Hips

How Do I Feel About
My Progress Today?

BREAKFAST			LUNCH		
TIME:			TIME:		
LOCATION:			LOCATION:		
FOOD ITEM	CALORIES	CARBS	FOOD ITEM	CALORIES	CARBS
TOTAL:			TOTAL:		

DINNER			SNACK		
TIME:			TIME:		
LOCATION:			LOCATION:		
FOOD ITEM	CALORIES	CARBS	FOOD ITEM	CALORIES	CARBS
TOTAL:			TOTAL:		

Exercise Activity: Hours || Minutes || Calories Burned

Measurements: Weight || Chest || Waist || Hips

How Do I Feel About
My Progress Today?

BREAKFAST			LUNCH		
TIME:			TIME:		
LOCATION:			LOCATION:		
FOOD ITEM	CALORIES	CARBS	FOOD ITEM	CALORIES	CARBS
TOTAL:			TOTAL:		

DINNER			SNACK		
TIME:			TIME:		
LOCATION:			LOCATION:		
FOOD ITEM	CALORIES	CARBS	FOOD ITEM	CALORIES	CARBS
TOTAL:			TOTAL:		

Exercise Activity: Hours || Minutes || Calories Burned

Measurements: Weight || Chest || Waist || Hips

How Do I Feel About
My Progress Today?

BREAKFAST			LUNCH		
TIME:			TIME:		
LOCATION:			LOCATION:		
FOOD ITEM	CALORIES	CARBS	FOOD ITEM	CALORIES	CARBS
TOTAL:			TOTAL:		

DINNER			SNACK		
TIME:			TIME:		
LOCATION:			LOCATION:		
FOOD ITEM	CALORIES	CARBS	FOOD ITEM	CALORIES	CARBS
TOTAL:			TOTAL:		

Exercise Activity: Hours || Minutes || Calories Burned

Measurements: Weight || Chest || Waist || Hips

How Do I Feel About
My Progress Today?

BREAKFAST			LUNCH		
TIME:			TIME:		
LOCATION:			LOCATION:		
FOOD ITEM	CALORIES	CARBS	FOOD ITEM	CALORIES	CARBS
TOTAL:			TOTAL:		

DINNER			SNACK		
TIME:			TIME:		
LOCATION:			LOCATION:		
FOOD ITEM	CALORIES	CARBS	FOOD ITEM	CALORIES	CARBS
TOTAL:			TOTAL:		

DATE _____

Exercise Activity: Hours || Minutes || Calories Burned

_____

Measurements: Weight || Chest || Waist || Hips

_____

How Do I Feel About
My Progress Today?

BREAKFAST			LUNCH		
TIME:			TIME:		
LOCATION:			LOCATION:		
FOOD ITEM	CALORIES	CARBS	FOOD ITEM	CALORIES	CARBS
TOTAL:			TOTAL:		

DINNER			SNACK		
TIME:			TIME:		
LOCATION:			LOCATION:		
FOOD ITEM	CALORIES	CARBS	FOOD ITEM	CALORIES	CARBS
TOTAL:			TOTAL:		

DATE _____

Exercise Activity: Hours ‖ Minutes ‖ Calories Burned

Measurements: Weight ‖ Chest ‖ Waist ‖ Hips

How Do I Feel About
My Progress Today?

BREAKFAST			LUNCH		
TIME:			TIME:		
LOCATION:			LOCATION:		
FOOD ITEM	CALORIES	CARBS	FOOD ITEM	CALORIES	CARBS
TOTAL:			TOTAL:		

DINNER			SNACK		
TIME:			TIME:		
LOCATION:			LOCATION:		
FOOD ITEM	CALORIES	CARBS	FOOD ITEM	CALORIES	CARBS
TOTAL:			TOTAL:		

Exercise Activity: Hours || Minutes || Calories Burned

Measurements: Weight || Chest || Waist || Hips

How Do I Feel About My Progress Today?

BREAKFAST			LUNCH		
TIME:			TIME:		
LOCATION:			LOCATION:		
FOOD ITEM	CALORIES	CARBS	FOOD ITEM	CALORIES	CARBS
TOTAL:			TOTAL:		

DINNER			SNACK		
TIME:			TIME:		
LOCATION:			LOCATION:		
FOOD ITEM	CALORIES	CARBS	FOOD ITEM	CALORIES	CARBS
TOTAL:			TOTAL:		

Exercise Activity: Hours || Minutes || Calories Burned

Measurements: Weight || Chest || Waist || Hips

How Do I Feel About
My Progress Today?

BREAKFAST			LUNCH		
TIME:			TIME:		
LOCATION:			LOCATION:		
FOOD ITEM	CALORIES	CARBS	FOOD ITEM	CALORIES	CARBS
TOTAL:			TOTAL:		

DINNER			SNACK		
TIME:			TIME:		
LOCATION:			LOCATION:		
FOOD ITEM	CALORIES	CARBS	FOOD ITEM	CALORIES	CARBS
TOTAL:			TOTAL:		

DATE _____

Exercise Activity: Hours || Minutes || Calories Burned

Measurements: Weight || Chest || Waist || Hips

How Do I Feel About My Progress Today?

BREAKFAST			LUNCH		
TIME:			TIME:		
LOCATION:			LOCATION:		
FOOD ITEM	CALORIES	CARBS	FOOD ITEM	CALORIES	CARBS
TOTAL:			TOTAL:		

DINNER			SNACK		
TIME:			TIME:		
LOCATION:			LOCATION:		
FOOD ITEM	CALORIES	CARBS	FOOD ITEM	CALORIES	CARBS
TOTAL:			TOTAL:		

Exercise Activity: Hours ‖ Minutes ‖ Calories Burned

Measurements: Weight ‖ Chest ‖ Waist ‖ Hips

How Do I Feel About
My Progress Today?

BREAKFAST			LUNCH		
TIME:			TIME:		
LOCATION:			LOCATION:		
FOOD ITEM	CALORIES	CARBS	FOOD ITEM	CALORIES	CARBS
TOTAL:			TOTAL:		
DINNER			SNACK		
TIME:			TIME:		
LOCATION:			LOCATION:		
FOOD ITEM	CALORIES	CARBS	FOOD ITEM	CALORIES	CARBS
TOTAL:			TOTAL:		

DATE _____

Exercise Activity: Hours || Minutes || Calories Burned

_____

Measurements: Weight || Chest || Waist || Hips

_____

How Do I Feel About
My Progress Today?

BREAKFAST			LUNCH		
TIME:			TIME:		
LOCATION:			LOCATION:		
FOOD ITEM	CALORIES	CARBS	FOOD ITEM	CALORIES	CARBS
TOTAL:			TOTAL:		

DINNER			SNACK		
TIME:			TIME:		
LOCATION:			LOCATION:		
FOOD ITEM	CALORIES	CARBS	FOOD ITEM	CALORIES	CARBS
TOTAL:			TOTAL:		

Exercise Activity: Hours || Minutes || Calories Burned

Measurements: Weight || Chest || Waist || Hips

How Do I Feel About
My Progress Today?

BREAKFAST			LUNCH		
TIME:			TIME:		
LOCATION:			LOCATION:		
FOOD ITEM	CALORIES	CARBS	FOOD ITEM	CALORIES	CARBS
TOTAL:			TOTAL:		

DINNER			SNACK		
TIME:			TIME:		
LOCATION:			LOCATION:		
FOOD ITEM	CALORIES	CARBS	FOOD ITEM	CALORIES	CARBS
TOTAL:			TOTAL:		

DATE _____

Exercise Activity: Hours || Minutes || Calories Burned

Measurements: Weight || Chest || Waist || Hips

How Do I Feel About
My Progress Today?

BREAKFAST				LUNCH			
TIME:				TIME:			
LOCATION:				LOCATION:			
FOOD ITEM		CALORIES	CARBS	FOOD ITEM		CALORIES	CARBS
TOTAL:				TOTAL:			

DINNER				SNACK			
TIME:				TIME:			
LOCATION:				LOCATION:			
FOOD ITEM		CALORIES	CARBS	FOOD ITEM		CALORIES	CARBS
TOTAL:				TOTAL:			

DATE _____

Exercise Activity: Hours || Minutes || Calories Burned

Measurements: Weight || Chest || Waist || Hips

How Do I Feel About
My Progress Today?

BREAKFAST			LUNCH		
TIME:			TIME:		
LOCATION:			LOCATION:		
FOOD ITEM	CALORIES	CARBS	FOOD ITEM	CALORIES	CARBS
TOTAL:			TOTAL:		

DINNER			SNACK		
TIME:			TIME:		
LOCATION:			LOCATION:		
FOOD ITEM	CALORIES	CARBS	FOOD ITEM	CALORIES	CARBS
TOTAL:			TOTAL:		

DATE _____

Exercise Activity: Hours || Minutes || Calories Burned

Measurements: Weight || Chest || Waist || Hips

How Do I Feel About My Progress Today?

BREAKFAST			LUNCH		
TIME:			TIME:		
LOCATION:			LOCATION:		
FOOD ITEM	CALORIES	CARBS	FOOD ITEM	CALORIES	CARBS
TOTAL:			TOTAL:		

DINNER			SNACK		
TIME:			TIME:		
LOCATION:			LOCATION:		
FOOD ITEM	CALORIES	CARBS	FOOD ITEM	CALORIES	CARBS
TOTAL:			TOTAL:		

DATE _____

Exercise Activity: Hours || Minutes || Calories Burned

_____

Measurements: Weight || Chest || Waist || Hips

_____

How Do I Feel About
My Progress Today?

BREAKFAST			LUNCH		
TIME:			TIME:		
LOCATION:			LOCATION:		
FOOD ITEM	CALORIES	CARBS	FOOD ITEM	CALORIES	CARBS
TOTAL:			TOTAL:		

DINNER			SNACK		
TIME:			TIME:		
LOCATION:			LOCATION:		
FOOD ITEM	CALORIES	CARBS	FOOD ITEM	CALORIES	CARBS
TOTAL:			TOTAL:		

DATE _____

Exercise Activity: Hours || Minutes || Calories Burned

Measurements: Weight || Chest || Waist || Hips

How Do I Feel About
My Progress Today?

BREAKFAST			LUNCH		
TIME:			TIME:		
LOCATION:			LOCATION:		
FOOD ITEM	CALORIES	CARBS	FOOD ITEM	CALORIES	CARBS
TOTAL:			TOTAL:		

DINNER			SNACK		
TIME:			TIME:		
LOCATION:			LOCATION:		
FOOD ITEM	CALORIES	CARBS	FOOD ITEM	CALORIES	CARBS
TOTAL:			TOTAL:		

DATE _____

Exercise Activity: Hours ‖ Minutes ‖ Calories Burned

Measurements: Weight ‖ Chest ‖ Waist ‖ Hips

How Do I Feel About My Progress Today?

BREAKFAST			LUNCH		
TIME:			TIME:		
LOCATION:			LOCATION:		
FOOD ITEM	CALORIES	CARBS	FOOD ITEM	CALORIES	CARBS
TOTAL:			TOTAL:		

DINNER			SNACK		
TIME:			TIME:		
LOCATION:			LOCATION:		
FOOD ITEM	CALORIES	CARBS	FOOD ITEM	CALORIES	CARBS
TOTAL:			TOTAL:		

DATE _____

Exercise Activity: Hours || Minutes || Calories Burned

Measurements: Weight || Chest || Waist || Hips

How Do I Feel About
My Progress Today?

BREAKFAST				LUNCH			
TIME:				TIME:			
LOCATION:				LOCATION:			
FOOD ITEM		CALORIES	CARBS	FOOD ITEM		CALORIES	CARBS
TOTAL:				TOTAL:			

DINNER				SNACK			
TIME:				TIME:			
LOCATION:				LOCATION:			
FOOD ITEM		CALORIES	CARBS	FOOD ITEM		CALORIES	CARBS
TOTAL:				TOTAL:			

Exercise Activity: Hours || Minutes || Calories Burned

Measurements: Weight || Chest || Waist || Hips

How Do I Feel About
My Progress Today?

BREAKFAST			LUNCH		
TIME:			TIME:		
LOCATION:			LOCATION:		
FOOD ITEM	CALORIES	CARBS	FOOD ITEM	CALORIES	CARBS
TOTAL:			TOTAL:		

DINNER			SNACK		
TIME:			TIME:		
LOCATION:			LOCATION:		
FOOD ITEM	CALORIES	CARBS	FOOD ITEM	CALORIES	CARBS
TOTAL:			TOTAL:		

DATE _____

Exercise Activity: Hours || Minutes || Calories Burned

Measurements: Weight || Chest || Waist || Hips

How Do I Feel About
My Progress Today?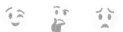

BREAKFAST				LUNCH			
TIME:				TIME:			
LOCATION:				LOCATION:			
FOOD ITEM		CALORIES	CARBS	FOOD ITEM		CALORIES	CARBS
TOTAL:				TOTAL:			

DINNER				SNACK			
TIME:				TIME:			
LOCATION:				LOCATION:			
FOOD ITEM		CALORIES	CARBS	FOOD ITEM		CALORIES	CARBS
TOTAL:				TOTAL:			

Exercise Activity: Hours ‖ Minutes ‖ Calories Burned

Measurements: Weight ‖ Chest ‖ Waist ‖ Hips

How Do I Feel About My Progress Today?

BREAKFAST			LUNCH		
TIME:			TIME:		
LOCATION:			LOCATION:		
FOOD ITEM	CALORIES	CARBS	FOOD ITEM	CALORIES	CARBS
TOTAL:			TOTAL:		

DINNER			SNACK		
TIME:			TIME:		
LOCATION:			LOCATION:		
FOOD ITEM	CALORIES	CARBS	FOOD ITEM	CALORIES	CARBS
TOTAL:			TOTAL:		

DATE _____

Exercise Activity: Hours ‖ Minutes ‖ Calories Burned

Measurements: Weight ‖ Chest ‖ Waist ‖ Hips

How Do I Feel About
My Progress Today?

BREAKFAST				LUNCH			
TIME:				TIME:			
LOCATION:				LOCATION:			
FOOD ITEM		CALORIES	CARBS	FOOD ITEM		CALORIES	CARBS
TOTAL:				TOTAL:			

DINNER				SNACK			
TIME:				TIME:			
LOCATION:				LOCATION:			
FOOD ITEM		CALORIES	CARBS	FOOD ITEM		CALORIES	CARBS
TOTAL:				TOTAL:			

DATE _____

Exercise Activity: Hours || Minutes || Calories Burned

Measurements: Weight || Chest || Waist || Hips

How Do I Feel About
My Progress Today?

BREAKFAST			LUNCH		
TIME:			TIME:		
LOCATION:			LOCATION:		
FOOD ITEM	CALORIES	CARBS	FOOD ITEM	CALORIES	CARBS
TOTAL:			TOTAL:		

DINNER			SNACK		
TIME:			TIME:		
LOCATION:			LOCATION:		
FOOD ITEM	CALORIES	CARBS	FOOD ITEM	CALORIES	CARBS
TOTAL:			TOTAL:		

DATE _____

Exercise Activity: Hours || Minutes || Calories Burned

Measurements: Weight || Chest || Waist || Hips

How Do I Feel About
My Progress Today?

BREAKFAST				LUNCH		
TIME:				TIME:		
LOCATION:				LOCATION:		
FOOD ITEM		CALORIES	CARBS	FOOD ITEM		CALORIES	CARBS
TOTAL:				TOTAL:		

DINNER				SNACK		
TIME:				TIME:		
LOCATION:				LOCATION:		
FOOD ITEM		CALORIES	CARBS	FOOD ITEM		CALORIES	CARBS
TOTAL:				TOTAL:		

Exercise Activity: Hours || Minutes || Calories Burned

Measurements: Weight || Chest || Waist || Hips

How Do I Feel About
My Progress Today?

BREAKFAST			LUNCH		
TIME:			TIME:		
LOCATION:			LOCATION:		
FOOD ITEM	CALORIES	CARBS	FOOD ITEM	CALORIES	CARBS
TOTAL:			TOTAL:		

DINNER			SNACK		
TIME:			TIME:		
LOCATION:			LOCATION:		
FOOD ITEM	CALORIES	CARBS	FOOD ITEM	CALORIES	CARBS
TOTAL:			TOTAL:		

DATE _____

Exercise Activity: Hours || Minutes || Calories Burned

Measurements: Weight || Chest || Waist || Hips

How Do I Feel About My Progress Today?

BREAKFAST			LUNCH		
TIME:			TIME:		
LOCATION:			LOCATION:		
FOOD ITEM	CALORIES	CARBS	FOOD ITEM	CALORIES	CARBS
TOTAL:			TOTAL:		

DINNER			SNACK		
TIME:			TIME:		
LOCATION:			LOCATION:		
FOOD ITEM	CALORIES	CARBS	FOOD ITEM	CALORIES	CARBS
TOTAL:			TOTAL:		

DATE _____

Exercise Activity: Hours ‖ Minutes ‖ Calories Burned

Measurements: Weight ‖ Chest ‖ Waist ‖ Hips

How Do I Feel About
My Progress Today?

BREAKFAST			LUNCH		
TIME:			TIME:		
LOCATION:			LOCATION:		
FOOD ITEM	CALORIES	CARBS	FOOD ITEM	CALORIES	CARBS
TOTAL:			TOTAL:		

DINNER			SNACK		
TIME:			TIME:		
LOCATION:			LOCATION:		
FOOD ITEM	CALORIES	CARBS	FOOD ITEM	CALORIES	CARBS
TOTAL:			TOTAL:		

DATE _____

Exercise Activity: Hours || Minutes || Calories Burned

_____

Measurements: Weight || Chest || Waist || Hips

_____

How Do I Feel About My Progress Today?

BREAKFAST			LUNCH		
TIME:			TIME:		
LOCATION:			LOCATION:		
FOOD ITEM	CALORIES	CARBS	FOOD ITEM	CALORIES	CARBS
TOTAL:			TOTAL:		

DINNER			SNACK		
TIME:			TIME:		
LOCATION:			LOCATION:		
FOOD ITEM	CALORIES	CARBS	FOOD ITEM	CALORIES	CARBS
TOTAL:			TOTAL:		

DATE _____

Exercise Activity: Hours || Minutes || Calories Burned

Measurements: Weight || Chest || Waist || Hips

How Do I Feel About
My Progress Today?

BREAKFAST			LUNCH		
TIME:			TIME:		
LOCATION:			LOCATION:		
FOOD ITEM	CALORIES	CARBS	FOOD ITEM	CALORIES	CARBS
TOTAL:			TOTAL:		

DINNER			SNACK		
TIME:			TIME:		
LOCATION:			LOCATION:		
FOOD ITEM	CALORIES	CARBS	FOOD ITEM	CALORIES	CARBS
TOTAL:			TOTAL:		

DATE _____

Exercise Activity: Hours || Minutes || Calories Burned

Measurements: Weight || Chest || Waist || Hips

How Do I Feel About
My Progress Today?

BREAKFAST			LUNCH		
TIME:			TIME:		
LOCATION:			LOCATION:		
FOOD ITEM	CALORIES	CARBS	FOOD ITEM	CALORIES	CARBS
TOTAL:			TOTAL:		

DINNER			SNACK		
TIME:			TIME:		
LOCATION:			LOCATION:		
FOOD ITEM	CALORIES	CARBS	FOOD ITEM	CALORIES	CARBS
TOTAL:			TOTAL:		

Exercise Activity: Hours || Minutes || Calories Burned

Measurements: Weight || Chest || Waist || Hips

How Do I Feel About
My Progress Today?

BREAKFAST			LUNCH		
TIME:			TIME:		
LOCATION:			LOCATION:		
FOOD ITEM	CALORIES	CARBS	FOOD ITEM	CALORIES	CARBS
TOTAL:			TOTAL:		

DINNER			SNACK		
TIME:			TIME:		
LOCATION:			LOCATION:		
FOOD ITEM	CALORIES	CARBS	FOOD ITEM	CALORIES	CARBS
TOTAL:			TOTAL:		

Exercise Activity: Hours || Minutes || Calories Burned

Measurements: Weight || Chest || Waist || Hips

How Do I Feel About
My Progress Today?

BREAKFAST			LUNCH		
TIME:			TIME:		
LOCATION:			LOCATION:		
FOOD ITEM	CALORIES	CARBS	FOOD ITEM	CALORIES	CARBS
TOTAL:			TOTAL:		

DINNER			SNACK		
TIME:			TIME:		
LOCATION:			LOCATION:		
FOOD ITEM	CALORIES	CARBS	FOOD ITEM	CALORIES	CARBS
TOTAL:			TOTAL:		

DATE _____

Exercise Activity: Hours || Minutes || Calories Burned

Measurements: Weight || Chest || Waist || Hips

How Do I Feel About
My Progress Today?

BREAKFAST			LUNCH		
TIME:			TIME:		
LOCATION:			LOCATION:		
FOOD ITEM	CALORIES	CARBS	FOOD ITEM	CALORIES	CARBS
TOTAL:			TOTAL:		

DINNER			SNACK		
TIME:			TIME:		
LOCATION:			LOCATION:		
FOOD ITEM	CALORIES	CARBS	FOOD ITEM	CALORIES	CARBS
TOTAL:			TOTAL:		

DATE _____

Exercise Activity: Hours ‖ Minutes ‖ Calories Burned

Measurements: Weight ‖ Chest ‖ Waist ‖ Hips

How Do I Feel About
My Progress Today?

BREAKFAST			LUNCH		
TIME:			TIME:		
LOCATION:			LOCATION:		
FOOD ITEM	CALORIES	CARBS	FOOD ITEM	CALORIES	CARBS
TOTAL:			TOTAL:		

DINNER			SNACK		
TIME:			TIME:		
LOCATION:			LOCATION:		
FOOD ITEM	CALORIES	CARBS	FOOD ITEM	CALORIES	CARBS
TOTAL:			TOTAL:		

DATE _____

Exercise Activity: Hours ‖ Minutes ‖ Calories Burned

Measurements: Weight ‖ Chest ‖ Waist ‖ Hips

How Do I Feel About
My Progress Today?

BREAKFAST			LUNCH		
TIME:			TIME:		
LOCATION:			LOCATION:		
FOOD ITEM	CALORIES	CARBS	FOOD ITEM	CALORIES	CARBS
TOTAL:			TOTAL:		

DINNER			SNACK		
TIME:			TIME:		
LOCATION:			LOCATION:		
FOOD ITEM	CALORIES	CARBS	FOOD ITEM	CALORIES	CARBS
TOTAL:			TOTAL:		

DATE _____

Exercise Activity: Hours || Minutes || Calories Burned

Measurements: Weight || Chest || Waist || Hips

How Do I Feel About My Progress Today?

BREAKFAST			LUNCH		
TIME:			TIME:		
LOCATION:			LOCATION:		
FOOD ITEM	CALORIES	CARBS	FOOD ITEM	CALORIES	CARBS
TOTAL:			TOTAL:		

DINNER			SNACK		
TIME:			TIME:		
LOCATION:			LOCATION:		
FOOD ITEM	CALORIES	CARBS	FOOD ITEM	CALORIES	CARBS
TOTAL:			TOTAL:		

DATE _____

Exercise Activity: Hours ‖ Minutes ‖ Calories Burned

_____

Measurements: Weight ‖ Chest ‖ Waist ‖ Hips

_____

How Do I Feel About
My Progress Today?

BREAKFAST			LUNCH		
TIME:			TIME:		
LOCATION:			LOCATION:		
FOOD ITEM	CALORIES	CARBS	FOOD ITEM	CALORIES	CARBS
TOTAL:			TOTAL:		

DINNER			SNACK		
TIME:			TIME:		
LOCATION:			LOCATION:		
FOOD ITEM	CALORIES	CARBS	FOOD ITEM	CALORIES	CARBS
TOTAL:			TOTAL:		

DATE _____

Exercise Activity: Hours ‖ Minutes ‖ Calories Burned

Measurements: Weight ‖ Chest ‖ Waist ‖ Hips

How Do I Feel About
My Progress Today?

BREAKFAST			LUNCH		
TIME:			TIME:		
LOCATION:			LOCATION:		
FOOD ITEM	CALORIES	CARBS	FOOD ITEM	CALORIES	CARBS
TOTAL:			TOTAL:		

DINNER			SNACK		
TIME:			TIME:		
LOCATION:			LOCATION:		
FOOD ITEM	CALORIES	CARBS	FOOD ITEM	CALORIES	CARBS
TOTAL:			TOTAL:		

Exercise Activity: Hours || Minutes || Calories Burned

Measurements: Weight || Chest || Waist || Hips

How Do I Feel About
My Progress Today?

BREAKFAST			LUNCH		
TIME:			TIME:		
LOCATION:			LOCATION:		
FOOD ITEM	CALORIES	CARBS	FOOD ITEM	CALORIES	CARBS
TOTAL:			TOTAL:		

DINNER			SNACK		
TIME:			TIME:		
LOCATION:			LOCATION:		
FOOD ITEM	CALORIES	CARBS	FOOD ITEM	CALORIES	CARBS
TOTAL:			TOTAL:		

Exercise Activity: Hours ‖ Minutes ‖ Calories Burned

Measurements: Weight ‖ Chest ‖ Waist ‖ Hips

How Do I Feel About
My Progress Today?

BREAKFAST			LUNCH		
TIME:			TIME:		
LOCATION:			LOCATION:		
FOOD ITEM	CALORIES	CARBS	FOOD ITEM	CALORIES	CARBS
TOTAL:			TOTAL:		

DINNER			SNACK		
TIME:			TIME:		
LOCATION:			LOCATION:		
FOOD ITEM	CALORIES	CARBS	FOOD ITEM	CALORIES	CARBS
TOTAL:			TOTAL:		

DATE _____

Exercise Activity: Hours || Minutes || Calories Burned

Measurements: Weight || Chest || Waist || Hips

How Do I Feel About
My Progress Today?

BREAKFAST			LUNCH		
TIME:			TIME:		
LOCATION:			LOCATION:		
FOOD ITEM	CALORIES	CARBS	FOOD ITEM	CALORIES	CARBS
TOTAL:			TOTAL:		

DINNER			SNACK		
TIME:			TIME:		
LOCATION:			LOCATION:		
FOOD ITEM	CALORIES	CARBS	FOOD ITEM	CALORIES	CARBS
TOTAL:			TOTAL:		

DATE _____

Exercise Activity: Hours || Minutes || Calories Burned

Measurements: Weight || Chest || Waist || Hips

How Do I Feel About My Progress Today?

BREAKFAST				LUNCH			
TIME:				TIME:			
LOCATION:				LOCATION:			
FOOD ITEM		CALORIES	CARBS	FOOD ITEM		CALORIES	CARBS
TOTAL:				TOTAL:			

DINNER				SNACK			
TIME:				TIME:			
LOCATION:				LOCATION:			
FOOD ITEM		CALORIES	CARBS	FOOD ITEM		CALORIES	CARBS
TOTAL:				TOTAL:			

DATE _____

Exercise Activity: Hours || Minutes || Calories Burned

Measurements: Weight || Chest || Waist || Hips

How Do I Feel About My Progress Today?

BREAKFAST			LUNCH		
TIME:			TIME:		
LOCATION:			LOCATION:		
FOOD ITEM	CALORIES	CARBS	FOOD ITEM	CALORIES	CARBS
TOTAL:			TOTAL:		

DINNER			SNACK		
TIME:			TIME:		
LOCATION:			LOCATION:		
FOOD ITEM	CALORIES	CARBS	FOOD ITEM	CALORIES	CARBS
TOTAL:			TOTAL:		

DATE _____

Exercise Activity: Hours || Minutes || Calories Burned

Measurements: Weight || Chest || Waist || Hips

How Do I Feel About
My Progress Today?

BREAKFAST			LUNCH		
TIME:			TIME:		
LOCATION:			LOCATION:		
FOOD ITEM	CALORIES	CARBS	FOOD ITEM	CALORIES	CARBS
TOTAL:			TOTAL:		

DINNER			SNACK		
TIME:			TIME:		
LOCATION:			LOCATION:		
FOOD ITEM	CALORIES	CARBS	FOOD ITEM	CALORIES	CARBS
TOTAL:			TOTAL:		

DATE _____

Exercise Activity: Hours ‖ Minutes ‖ Calories Burned

_____

Measurements: Weight ‖ Chest ‖ Waist ‖ Hips

_____

How Do I Feel About
My Progress Today?

BREAKFAST			LUNCH		
TIME:			TIME:		
LOCATION:			LOCATION:		
FOOD ITEM	CALORIES	CARBS	FOOD ITEM	CALORIES	CARBS
TOTAL:			TOTAL:		

DINNER			SNACK		
TIME:			TIME:		
LOCATION:			LOCATION:		
FOOD ITEM	CALORIES	CARBS	FOOD ITEM	CALORIES	CARBS
TOTAL:			TOTAL:		

DATE _____

Exercise Activity: Hours ‖ Minutes ‖ Calories Burned

Measurements: Weight ‖ Chest ‖ Waist ‖ Hips

How Do I Feel About
My Progress Today?

BREAKFAST			LUNCH		
TIME:			TIME:		
LOCATION:			LOCATION:		
FOOD ITEM	CALORIES	CARBS	FOOD ITEM	CALORIES	CARBS
TOTAL:			TOTAL:		

DINNER			SNACK		
TIME:			TIME:		
LOCATION:			LOCATION:		
FOOD ITEM	CALORIES	CARBS	FOOD ITEM	CALORIES	CARBS
TOTAL:			TOTAL:		

Exercise Activity: Hours || Minutes || Calories Burned

Measurements: Weight || Chest || Waist || Hips

How Do I Feel About
My Progress Today?

BREAKFAST			**LUNCH**		
TIME:			TIME:		
LOCATION:			LOCATION:		
FOOD ITEM	CALORIES	CARBS	FOOD ITEM	CALORIES	CARBS
TOTAL:			TOTAL:		
DINNER			**SNACK**		
TIME:			TIME:		
LOCATION:			LOCATION:		
FOOD ITEM	CALORIES	CARBS	FOOD ITEM	CALORIES	CARBS
TOTAL:			TOTAL:		

DATE _____

Exercise Activity: Hours || Minutes || Calories Burned

Measurements: Weight || Chest || Waist || Hips

How Do I Feel About
My Progress Today?   😄   😉   🤔   🙁   😣

BREAKFAST		
TIME:		
LOCATION:		
FOOD ITEM	CALORIES	CARBS
TOTAL:		

LUNCH		
TIME:		
LOCATION:		
FOOD ITEM	CALORIES	CARBS
TOTAL:		

DINNER		
TIME:		
LOCATION:		
FOOD ITEM	CALORIES	CARBS
TOTAL:		

SNACK		
TIME:		
LOCATION:		
FOOD ITEM	CALORIES	CARBS
TOTAL:		

Exercise Activity: Hours || Minutes || Calories Burned

Measurements: Weight || Chest || Waist || Hips

How Do I Feel About
My Progress Today?

BREAKFAST			LUNCH		
TIME:			TIME:		
LOCATION:			LOCATION:		
FOOD ITEM	CALORIES	CARBS	FOOD ITEM	CALORIES	CARBS
TOTAL:			TOTAL:		

DINNER			SNACK		
TIME:			TIME:		
LOCATION:			LOCATION:		
FOOD ITEM	CALORIES	CARBS	FOOD ITEM	CALORIES	CARBS
TOTAL:			TOTAL:		

DATE _____

Exercise Activity: Hours || Minutes || Calories Burned

Measurements: Weight || Chest || Waist || Hips

How Do I Feel About
My Progress Today?

BREAKFAST			LUNCH		
TIME:			TIME:		
LOCATION:			LOCATION:		
FOOD ITEM	CALORIES	CARBS	FOOD ITEM	CALORIES	CARBS
TOTAL:			TOTAL:		

DINNER			SNACK		
TIME:			TIME:		
LOCATION:			LOCATION:		
FOOD ITEM	CALORIES	CARBS	FOOD ITEM	CALORIES	CARBS
TOTAL:			TOTAL:		

Exercise Activity: Hours || Minutes || Calories Burned

Measurements: Weight || Chest || Waist || Hips

How Do I Feel About My Progress Today?

BREAKFAST			LUNCH		
TIME:			TIME:		
LOCATION:			LOCATION:		
FOOD ITEM	CALORIES	CARBS	FOOD ITEM	CALORIES	CARBS
TOTAL:			TOTAL:		

DINNER			SNACK		
TIME:			TIME:		
LOCATION:			LOCATION:		
FOOD ITEM	CALORIES	CARBS	FOOD ITEM	CALORIES	CARBS
TOTAL:			TOTAL:		

DATE _____

Exercise Activity: Hours || Minutes || Calories Burned

Measurements: Weight || Chest || Waist || Hips

How Do I Feel About
My Progress Today?

BREAKFAST			LUNCH		
TIME:			TIME:		
LOCATION:			LOCATION:		
FOOD ITEM	CALORIES	CARBS	FOOD ITEM	CALORIES	CARBS
TOTAL:			TOTAL:		

DINNER			SNACK		
TIME:			TIME:		
LOCATION:			LOCATION:		
FOOD ITEM	CALORIES	CARBS	FOOD ITEM	CALORIES	CARBS
TOTAL:			TOTAL:		

DATE _____

Exercise Activity: Hours || Minutes || Calories Burned

Measurements: Weight || Chest || Waist || Hips

How Do I Feel About
My Progress Today?

BREAKFAST			LUNCH		
TIME:			TIME:		
LOCATION:			LOCATION:		
FOOD ITEM	CALORIES	CARBS	FOOD ITEM	CALORIES	CARBS
TOTAL:			TOTAL:		

DINNER			SNACK		
TIME:			TIME:		
LOCATION:			LOCATION:		
FOOD ITEM	CALORIES	CARBS	FOOD ITEM	CALORIES	CARBS
TOTAL:			TOTAL:		

_____

Exercise Activity: Hours || Minutes || Calories Burned

_____

Measurements: Weight || Chest || Waist || Hips

_____

How Do I Feel About
My Progress Today?

BREAKFAST			LUNCH		
TIME:			TIME:		
LOCATION:			LOCATION:		
FOOD ITEM	CALORIES	CARBS	FOOD ITEM	CALORIES	CARBS
TOTAL:			TOTAL:		

DINNER			SNACK		
TIME:			TIME:		
LOCATION:			LOCATION:		
FOOD ITEM	CALORIES	CARBS	FOOD ITEM	CALORIES	CARBS
TOTAL:			TOTAL:		

DATE _____

Exercise Activity: Hours ‖ Minutes ‖ Calories Burned

Measurements: Weight ‖ Chest ‖ Waist ‖ Hips

How Do I Feel About
My Progress Today?

BREAKFAST			LUNCH		
TIME:			TIME:		
LOCATION:			LOCATION:		
FOOD ITEM	CALORIES	CARBS	FOOD ITEM	CALORIES	CARBS
TOTAL:			TOTAL:		

DINNER			SNACK		
TIME:			TIME:		
LOCATION:			LOCATION:		
FOOD ITEM	CALORIES	CARBS	FOOD ITEM	CALORIES	CARBS
TOTAL:			TOTAL:		

DATE _____

Exercise Activity: Hours || Minutes || Calories Burned

Measurements: Weight || Chest || Waist || Hips

How Do I Feel About
My Progress Today?

BREAKFAST				LUNCH		
TIME:				TIME:		
LOCATION:				LOCATION:		
FOOD ITEM		CALORIES	CARBS	FOOD ITEM		CALORIES	CARBS
TOTAL:				TOTAL:		

DINNER				SNACK		
TIME:				TIME:		
LOCATION:				LOCATION:		
FOOD ITEM		CALORIES	CARBS	FOOD ITEM		CALORIES	CARBS
TOTAL:				TOTAL:		

DATE _____

Exercise Activity: Hours || Minutes || Calories Burned

Measurements: Weight || Chest || Waist || Hips

How Do I Feel About
My Progress Today?

BREAKFAST			LUNCH		
TIME:			TIME:		
LOCATION:			LOCATION:		
FOOD ITEM	CALORIES	CARBS	FOOD ITEM	CALORIES	CARBS
TOTAL:			TOTAL:		

DINNER			SNACK		
TIME:			TIME:		
LOCATION:			LOCATION:		
FOOD ITEM	CALORIES	CARBS	FOOD ITEM	CALORIES	CARBS
TOTAL:			TOTAL:		

DATE _____

Exercise Activity:　Hours　||　Minutes　||　Calories Burned

Measurements: Weight　||　Chest　||　Waist　||　Hips

How Do I Feel About
My Progress Today?

BREAKFAST				LUNCH		
TIME:				TIME:		
LOCATION:				LOCATION:		
FOOD ITEM		CALORIES	CARBS	FOOD ITEM		CALORIES	CARBS
TOTAL:				TOTAL:		

DINNER				SNACK		
TIME:				TIME:		
LOCATION:				LOCATION:		
FOOD ITEM		CALORIES	CARBS	FOOD ITEM		CALORIES	CARBS
TOTAL:				TOTAL:		

DATE _____

Exercise Activity: Hours || Minutes || Calories Burned

Measurements: Weight || Chest || Waist || Hips

How Do I Feel About
My Progress Today?

BREAKFAST			LUNCH		
TIME:			TIME:		
LOCATION:			LOCATION:		
FOOD ITEM	CALORIES	CARBS	FOOD ITEM	CALORIES	CARBS
TOTAL:			TOTAL:		

DINNER			SNACK		
TIME:			TIME:		
LOCATION:			LOCATION:		
FOOD ITEM	CALORIES	CARBS	FOOD ITEM	CALORIES	CARBS
TOTAL:			TOTAL:		

Exercise Activity: Hours || Minutes || Calories Burned

Measurements: Weight || Chest || Waist || Hips

How Do I Feel About
My Progress Today?

BREAKFAST			LUNCH		
TIME:			TIME:		
LOCATION:			LOCATION:		
FOOD ITEM	CALORIES	CARBS	FOOD ITEM	CALORIES	CARBS
TOTAL:			TOTAL:		

DINNER			SNACK		
TIME:			TIME:		
LOCATION:			LOCATION:		
FOOD ITEM	CALORIES	CARBS	FOOD ITEM	CALORIES	CARBS
TOTAL:			TOTAL:		

DATE _____

Exercise Activity: Hours || Minutes || Calories Burned

Measurements: Weight || Chest || Waist || Hips

How Do I Feel About My Progress Today?

BREAKFAST			LUNCH		
TIME:			TIME:		
LOCATION:			LOCATION:		
FOOD ITEM	CALORIES	CARBS	FOOD ITEM	CALORIES	CARBS
TOTAL:			TOTAL:		

DINNER			SNACK		
TIME:			TIME:		
LOCATION:			LOCATION:		
FOOD ITEM	CALORIES	CARBS	FOOD ITEM	CALORIES	CARBS
TOTAL:			TOTAL:		

DATE _____

Exercise Activity: Hours || Minutes || Calories Burned

Measurements: Weight || Chest || Waist || Hips

How Do I Feel About
My Progress Today?

BREAKFAST			LUNCH		
TIME:			TIME:		
LOCATION:			LOCATION:		
FOOD ITEM	CALORIES	CARBS	FOOD ITEM	CALORIES	CARBS
TOTAL:			TOTAL:		

DINNER			SNACK		
TIME:			TIME:		
LOCATION:			LOCATION:		
FOOD ITEM	CALORIES	CARBS	FOOD ITEM	CALORIES	CARBS
TOTAL:			TOTAL:		

DATE _____

Exercise Activity: Hours ‖ Minutes ‖ Calories Burned

Measurements: Weight ‖ Chest ‖ Waist ‖ Hips

How Do I Feel About
My Progress Today?

BREAKFAST			LUNCH		
TIME:			TIME:		
LOCATION:			LOCATION:		
FOOD ITEM	CALORIES	CARBS	FOOD ITEM	CALORIES	CARBS
TOTAL:			TOTAL:		
DINNER			**SNACK**		
TIME:			TIME:		
LOCATION:			LOCATION:		
FOOD ITEM	CALORIES	CARBS	FOOD ITEM	CALORIES	CARBS
TOTAL:			TOTAL:		

DATE _____

Exercise Activity: Hours ‖ Minutes ‖ Calories Burned

Measurements: Weight ‖ Chest ‖ Waist ‖ Hips

How Do I Feel About My Progress Today?

BREAKFAST			LUNCH		
TIME:			TIME:		
LOCATION:			LOCATION:		
FOOD ITEM	CALORIES	CARBS	FOOD ITEM	CALORIES	CARBS
TOTAL:			TOTAL:		

DINNER			SNACK		
TIME:			TIME:		
LOCATION:			LOCATION:		
FOOD ITEM	CALORIES	CARBS	FOOD ITEM	CALORIES	CARBS
TOTAL:			TOTAL:		

Exercise Activity: Hours || Minutes || Calories Burned

Measurements: Weight || Chest || Waist || Hips

How Do I Feel About
My Progress Today?

BREAKFAST			LUNCH		
TIME:			TIME:		
LOCATION:			LOCATION:		
FOOD ITEM	CALORIES	CARBS	FOOD ITEM	CALORIES	CARBS
TOTAL:			TOTAL:		

DINNER			SNACK		
TIME:			TIME:		
LOCATION:			LOCATION:		
FOOD ITEM	CALORIES	CARBS	FOOD ITEM	CALORIES	CARBS
TOTAL:			TOTAL:		

DATE _____

Exercise Activity: Hours || Minutes || Calories Burned

Measurements: Weight || Chest || Waist || Hips

How Do I Feel About
My Progress Today?

BREAKFAST			LUNCH		
TIME:			TIME:		
LOCATION:			LOCATION:		
FOOD ITEM	CALORIES	CARBS	FOOD ITEM	CALORIES	CARBS
TOTAL:			TOTAL:		

DINNER			SNACK		
TIME:			TIME:		
LOCATION:			LOCATION:		
FOOD ITEM	CALORIES	CARBS	FOOD ITEM	CALORIES	CARBS
TOTAL:			TOTAL:		

Exercise Activity: Hours ‖ Minutes ‖ Calories Burned

Measurements: Weight ‖ Chest ‖ Waist ‖ Hips

How Do I Feel About
My Progress Today?

BREAKFAST			LUNCH		
TIME:			TIME:		
LOCATION:			LOCATION:		
FOOD ITEM	CALORIES	CARBS	FOOD ITEM	CALORIES	CARBS
TOTAL:			TOTAL:		

DINNER			SNACK		
TIME:			TIME:		
LOCATION:			LOCATION:		
FOOD ITEM	CALORIES	CARBS	FOOD ITEM	CALORIES	CARBS
TOTAL:			TOTAL:		

DATE _____

Exercise Activity: Hours || Minutes || Calories Burned

Measurements: Weight || Chest || Waist || Hips

How Do I Feel About
My Progress Today?

BREAKFAST			LUNCH		
TIME:			TIME:		
LOCATION:			LOCATION:		
FOOD ITEM	CALORIES	CARBS	FOOD ITEM	CALORIES	CARBS
TOTAL:			TOTAL:		
DINNER			**SNACK**		
TIME:			TIME:		
LOCATION:			LOCATION:		
FOOD ITEM	CALORIES	CARBS	FOOD ITEM	CALORIES	CARBS
TOTAL:			TOTAL:		

DATE _____

Exercise Activity: Hours || Minutes || Calories Burned

Measurements: Weight || Chest || Waist || Hips

How Do I Feel About
My Progress Today?

BREAKFAST			LUNCH		
TIME:			TIME:		
LOCATION:			LOCATION:		
FOOD ITEM	CALORIES	CARBS	FOOD ITEM	CALORIES	CARBS
TOTAL:			TOTAL:		

DINNER			SNACK		
TIME:			TIME:		
LOCATION:			LOCATION:		
FOOD ITEM	CALORIES	CARBS	FOOD ITEM	CALORIES	CARBS
TOTAL:			TOTAL:		

DATE _____

Exercise Activity: Hours || Minutes || Calories Burned

_____

Measurements: Weight || Chest || Waist || Hips

_____

How Do I Feel About
My Progress Today?

BREAKFAST			LUNCH		
TIME:			TIME:		
LOCATION:			LOCATION:		
FOOD ITEM	CALORIES	CARBS	FOOD ITEM	CALORIES	CARBS
TOTAL:			TOTAL:		

DINNER			SNACK		
TIME:			TIME:		
LOCATION:			LOCATION:		
FOOD ITEM	CALORIES	CARBS	FOOD ITEM	CALORIES	CARBS
TOTAL:			TOTAL:		

Exercise Activity: Hours || Minutes || Calories Burned

Measurements: Weight || Chest || Waist || Hips

How Do I Feel About
My Progress Today?

BREAKFAST			LUNCH		
TIME:			TIME:		
LOCATION:			LOCATION:		
FOOD ITEM	CALORIES	CARBS	FOOD ITEM	CALORIES	CARBS
TOTAL:			TOTAL:		

DINNER			SNACK		
TIME:			TIME:		
LOCATION:			LOCATION:		
FOOD ITEM	CALORIES	CARBS	FOOD ITEM	CALORIES	CARBS
TOTAL:			TOTAL:		

DATE _____

Exercise Activity: Hours || Minutes || Calories Burned

Measurements: Weight || Chest || Waist || Hips

How Do I Feel About
My Progress Today?

BREAKFAST			LUNCH		
TIME:			TIME:		
LOCATION:			LOCATION:		
FOOD ITEM	CALORIES	CARBS	FOOD ITEM	CALORIES	CARBS
TOTAL:			TOTAL:		

DINNER			SNACK		
TIME:			TIME:		
LOCATION:			LOCATION:		
FOOD ITEM	CALORIES	CARBS	FOOD ITEM	CALORIES	CARBS
TOTAL:			TOTAL:		

DATE _____

Exercise Activity: Hours || Minutes || Calories Burned

Measurements: Weight || Chest || Waist || Hips

How Do I Feel About
My Progress Today?

BREAKFAST			LUNCH		
TIME:			TIME:		
LOCATION:			LOCATION:		
FOOD ITEM	CALORIES	CARBS	FOOD ITEM	CALORIES	CARBS
TOTAL:			TOTAL:		

DINNER			SNACK		
TIME:			TIME:		
LOCATION:			LOCATION:		
FOOD ITEM	CALORIES	CARBS	FOOD ITEM	CALORIES	CARBS
TOTAL:			TOTAL:		

Exercise Activity: Hours || Minutes || Calories Burned

Measurements: Weight || Chest || Waist || Hips

How Do I Feel About
My Progress Today?

BREAKFAST			LUNCH		
TIME:			TIME:		
LOCATION:			LOCATION:		
FOOD ITEM	CALORIES	CARBS	FOOD ITEM	CALORIES	CARBS
TOTAL:			TOTAL:		

DINNER			SNACK		
TIME:			TIME:		
LOCATION:			LOCATION:		
FOOD ITEM	CALORIES	CARBS	FOOD ITEM	CALORIES	CARBS
TOTAL:			TOTAL:		

DATE _____

Exercise Activity: Hours || Minutes || Calories Burned

_____

Measurements: Weight || Chest || Waist || Hips

_____

How Do I Feel About
My Progress Today?

BREAKFAST			LUNCH		
TIME:			TIME:		
LOCATION:			LOCATION:		
FOOD ITEM	CALORIES	CARBS	FOOD ITEM	CALORIES	CARBS
TOTAL:			TOTAL:		

DINNER			SNACK		
TIME:			TIME:		
LOCATION:			LOCATION:		
FOOD ITEM	CALORIES	CARBS	FOOD ITEM	CALORIES	CARBS
TOTAL:			TOTAL:		

DATE _____

Exercise Activity: Hours ‖ Minutes ‖ Calories Burned

Measurements: Weight ‖ Chest ‖ Waist ‖ Hips

How Do I Feel About
My Progress Today?   😄   😉   🤔   😟   😫

BREAKFAST				LUNCH		
TIME:				TIME:		
LOCATION:				LOCATION:		
FOOD ITEM	CALORIES	CARBS		FOOD ITEM	CALORIES	CARBS
TOTAL:				TOTAL:		

DINNER				SNACK		
TIME:				TIME:		
LOCATION:				LOCATION:		
FOOD ITEM	CALORIES	CARBS		FOOD ITEM	CALORIES	CARBS
TOTAL:				TOTAL:		

DATE _____

Exercise Activity: Hours || Minutes || Calories Burned

Measurements: Weight || Chest || Waist || Hips

How Do I Feel About My Progress Today?

BREAKFAST		
TIME:		
LOCATION:		
FOOD ITEM	CALORIES	CARBS
TOTAL:		

LUNCH		
TIME:		
LOCATION:		
FOOD ITEM	CALORIES	CARBS
TOTAL:		

DINNER		
TIME:		
LOCATION:		
FOOD ITEM	CALORIES	CARBS
TOTAL:		

SNACK		
TIME:		
LOCATION:		
FOOD ITEM	CALORIES	CARBS
TOTAL:		

DATE _____

Exercise Activity: Hours || Minutes || Calories Burned

Measurements: Weight || Chest || Waist || Hips

How Do I Feel About
My Progress Today?

BREAKFAST			LUNCH		
TIME:			TIME:		
LOCATION:			LOCATION:		
FOOD ITEM	CALORIES	CARBS	FOOD ITEM	CALORIES	CARBS
TOTAL:			TOTAL:		

DINNER			SNACK		
TIME:			TIME:		
LOCATION:			LOCATION:		
FOOD ITEM	CALORIES	CARBS	FOOD ITEM	CALORIES	CARBS
TOTAL:			TOTAL:		

DATE	

Exercise Activity: Hours || Minutes || Calories Burned

Measurements: Weight || Chest || Waist || Hips

How Do I Feel About My Progress Today?

BREAKFAST

TIME:

LOCATION:

FOOD ITEM	CALORIES	CARBS
TOTAL:		

LUNCH

TIME:

LOCATION:

FOOD ITEM	CALORIES	CARBS
TOTAL:		

DINNER

TIME:

LOCATION:

FOOD ITEM	CALORIES	CARBS
TOTAL:		

SNACK

TIME:

LOCATION:

FOOD ITEM	CALORIES	CARBS
TOTAL:		

DATE _____

Exercise Activity: Hours || Minutes || Calories Burned

Measurements: Weight || Chest || Waist || Hips

How Do I Feel About
My Progress Today?

BREAKFAST				LUNCH			
TIME:				TIME:			
LOCATION:				LOCATION:			
FOOD ITEM		CALORIES	CARBS	FOOD ITEM		CALORIES	CARBS
TOTAL:				TOTAL:			

DINNER				SNACK			
TIME:				TIME:			
LOCATION:				LOCATION:			
FOOD ITEM		CALORIES	CARBS	FOOD ITEM		CALORIES	CARBS
TOTAL:				TOTAL:			

DATE _____

Exercise Activity: Hours || Minutes || Calories Burned

Measurements: Weight || Chest || Waist || Hips

How Do I Feel About
My Progress Today?

BREAKFAST			LUNCH		
TIME:			TIME:		
LOCATION:			LOCATION:		
FOOD ITEM	CALORIES	CARBS	FOOD ITEM	CALORIES	CARBS
TOTAL:			TOTAL:		
DINNER			SNACK		
TIME:			TIME:		
LOCATION:			LOCATION:		
FOOD ITEM	CALORIES	CARBS	FOOD ITEM	CALORIES	CARBS
TOTAL:			TOTAL:		

DATE _____

Exercise Activity: Hours ‖ Minutes ‖ Calories Burned

_____

Measurements: Weight ‖ Chest ‖ Waist ‖ Hips

_____

How Do I Feel About
My Progress Today?

BREAKFAST			LUNCH		
TIME:			TIME:		
LOCATION:			LOCATION:		
FOOD ITEM	CALORIES	CARBS	FOOD ITEM	CALORIES	CARBS
TOTAL:			TOTAL:		

DINNER			SNACK		
TIME:			TIME:		
LOCATION:			LOCATION:		
FOOD ITEM	CALORIES	CARBS	FOOD ITEM	CALORIES	CARBS
TOTAL:			TOTAL:		

Exercise Activity: Hours ‖ Minutes ‖ Calories Burned

Measurements: Weight ‖ Chest ‖ Waist ‖ Hips

How Do I Feel About My Progress Today?

BREAKFAST			LUNCH		
TIME:			TIME:		
LOCATION:			LOCATION:		
FOOD ITEM	CALORIES	CARBS	FOOD ITEM	CALORIES	CARBS
TOTAL:			TOTAL:		

DINNER			SNACK		
TIME:			TIME:		
LOCATION:			LOCATION:		
FOOD ITEM	CALORIES	CARBS	FOOD ITEM	CALORIES	CARBS
TOTAL:			TOTAL:		

DATE _____

Exercise Activity: Hours ‖ Minutes ‖ Calories Burned

Measurements: Weight ‖ Chest ‖ Waist ‖ Hips

How Do I Feel About My Progress Today?

BREAKFAST			LUNCH		
TIME:			TIME:		
LOCATION:			LOCATION:		
FOOD ITEM	CALORIES	CARBS	FOOD ITEM	CALORIES	CARBS
TOTAL:			TOTAL:		

DINNER			SNACK		
TIME:			TIME:		
LOCATION:			LOCATION:		
FOOD ITEM	CALORIES	CARBS	FOOD ITEM	CALORIES	CARBS
TOTAL:			TOTAL:		

Exercise Activity: Hours || Minutes || Calories Burned

Measurements: Weight || Chest || Waist || Hips

How Do I Feel About
My Progress Today?

BREAKFAST			**LUNCH**		
TIME:			TIME:		
LOCATION:			LOCATION:		
FOOD ITEM	CALORIES	CARBS	FOOD ITEM	CALORIES	CARBS
TOTAL:			TOTAL:		

DINNER			**SNACK**		
TIME:			TIME:		
LOCATION:			LOCATION:		
FOOD ITEM	CALORIES	CARBS	FOOD ITEM	CALORIES	CARBS
TOTAL:			TOTAL:		

DATE _____

Exercise Activity: Hours || Minutes || Calories Burned

Measurements: Weight || Chest || Waist || Hips

How Do I Feel About
My Progress Today?

BREAKFAST			LUNCH		
TIME:			TIME:		
LOCATION:			LOCATION:		
FOOD ITEM	CALORIES	CARBS	FOOD ITEM	CALORIES	CARBS
TOTAL:			TOTAL:		

DINNER			SNACK		
TIME:			TIME:		
LOCATION:			LOCATION:		
FOOD ITEM	CALORIES	CARBS	FOOD ITEM	CALORIES	CARBS
TOTAL:			TOTAL:		

DATE _____

Exercise Activity: Hours || Minutes || Calories Burned

Measurements: Weight || Chest || Waist || Hips

How Do I Feel About My Progress Today?

BREAKFAST			LUNCH		
TIME:			TIME:		
LOCATION:			LOCATION:		
FOOD ITEM	CALORIES	CARBS	FOOD ITEM	CALORIES	CARBS
TOTAL:			TOTAL:		

DINNER			SNACK		
TIME:			TIME:		
LOCATION:			LOCATION:		
FOOD ITEM	CALORIES	CARBS	FOOD ITEM	CALORIES	CARBS
TOTAL:			TOTAL:		

DATE _____

Exercise Activity: Hours || Minutes || Calories Burned

Measurements: Weight || Chest || Waist || Hips

How Do I Feel About
My Progress Today?

BREAKFAST			LUNCH		
TIME:			TIME:		
LOCATION:			LOCATION:		
FOOD ITEM	CALORIES	CARBS	FOOD ITEM	CALORIES	CARBS
TOTAL:			TOTAL:		

DINNER			SNACK		
TIME:			TIME:		
LOCATION:			LOCATION:		
FOOD ITEM	CALORIES	CARBS	FOOD ITEM	CALORIES	CARBS
TOTAL:			TOTAL:		

DATE _____

Exercise Activity: Hours || Minutes || Calories Burned

Measurements: Weight || Chest || Waist || Hips

How Do I Feel About
My Progress Today?

BREAKFAST			LUNCH		
TIME:			TIME:		
LOCATION:			LOCATION:		
FOOD ITEM	CALORIES	CARBS	FOOD ITEM	CALORIES	CARBS
TOTAL:			TOTAL:		

DINNER			SNACK		
TIME:			TIME:		
LOCATION:			LOCATION:		
FOOD ITEM	CALORIES	CARBS	FOOD ITEM	CALORIES	CARBS
TOTAL:			TOTAL:		

DATE _____

Exercise Activity: Hours || Minutes || Calories Burned

Measurements: Weight || Chest || Waist || Hips

How Do I Feel About My Progress Today?

BREAKFAST			LUNCH		
TIME:			TIME:		
LOCATION:			LOCATION:		
FOOD ITEM	CALORIES	CARBS	FOOD ITEM	CALORIES	CARBS
TOTAL:			TOTAL:		

DINNER			SNACK		
TIME:			TIME:		
LOCATION:			LOCATION:		
FOOD ITEM	CALORIES	CARBS	FOOD ITEM	CALORIES	CARBS
TOTAL:			TOTAL:		

Exercise Activity: Hours || Minutes || Calories Burned

Measurements: Weight || Chest || Waist || Hips

How Do I Feel About
My Progress Today?

BREAKFAST			LUNCH		
TIME:			TIME:		
LOCATION:			LOCATION:		
FOOD ITEM	CALORIES	CARBS	FOOD ITEM	CALORIES	CARBS
TOTAL:			TOTAL:		

DINNER			SNACK		
TIME:			TIME:		
LOCATION:			LOCATION:		
FOOD ITEM	CALORIES	CARBS	FOOD ITEM	CALORIES	CARBS
TOTAL:			TOTAL:		

DATE _____

Exercise Activity: Hours || Minutes || Calories Burned

Measurements: Weight || Chest || Waist || Hips

How Do I Feel About
My Progress Today?

BREAKFAST			LUNCH		
TIME:			TIME:		
LOCATION:			LOCATION:		
FOOD ITEM	CALORIES	CARBS	FOOD ITEM	CALORIES	CARBS
TOTAL:			TOTAL:		

DINNER			SNACK		
TIME:			TIME:		
LOCATION:			LOCATION:		
FOOD ITEM	CALORIES	CARBS	FOOD ITEM	CALORIES	CARBS
TOTAL:			TOTAL:		

DATE _____

Exercise Activity: Hours || Minutes || Calories Burned

Measurements: Weight || Chest || Waist || Hips

How Do I Feel About
My Progress Today?

BREAKFAST			LUNCH		
TIME:			TIME:		
LOCATION:			LOCATION:		
FOOD ITEM	CALORIES	CARBS	FOOD ITEM	CALORIES	CARBS
TOTAL:			TOTAL:		

DINNER			SNACK		
TIME:			TIME:		
LOCATION:			LOCATION:		
FOOD ITEM	CALORIES	CARBS	FOOD ITEM	CALORIES	CARBS
TOTAL:			TOTAL:		

DATE _____

Exercise Activity: Hours ‖ Minutes ‖ Calories Burned

Measurements: Weight ‖ Chest ‖ Waist ‖ Hips

How Do I Feel About
My Progress Today?

BREAKFAST			LUNCH		
TIME:			TIME:		
LOCATION:			LOCATION:		
FOOD ITEM	CALORIES	CARBS	FOOD ITEM	CALORIES	CARBS
TOTAL:			TOTAL:		

DINNER			SNACK		
TIME:			TIME:		
LOCATION:			LOCATION:		
FOOD ITEM	CALORIES	CARBS	FOOD ITEM	CALORIES	CARBS
TOTAL:			TOTAL:		

DATE _____

Exercise Activity: Hours || Minutes || Calories Burned

Measurements: Weight || Chest || Waist || Hips

How Do I Feel About My Progress Today?   😄   😉   🤔   😟   😣

BREAKFAST				LUNCH		
TIME:				TIME:		
LOCATION:				LOCATION:		
FOOD ITEM		CALORIES	CARBS	FOOD ITEM		CALORIES	CARBS
TOTAL:				TOTAL:		

DINNER				SNACK		
TIME:				TIME:		
LOCATION:				LOCATION:		
FOOD ITEM		CALORIES	CARBS	FOOD ITEM		CALORIES	CARBS
TOTAL:				TOTAL:		

DATE _____

Exercise Activity: Hours ‖ Minutes ‖ Calories Burned

Measurements: Weight ‖ Chest ‖ Waist ‖ Hips

How Do I Feel About My Progress Today?

BREAKFAST				LUNCH		
TIME:				TIME:		
LOCATION:				LOCATION:		
FOOD ITEM		CALORIES	CARBS	FOOD ITEM		CALORIES	CARBS
TOTAL:				TOTAL:		

DINNER				SNACK		
TIME:				TIME:		
LOCATION:				LOCATION:		
FOOD ITEM		CALORIES	CARBS	FOOD ITEM		CALORIES	CARBS
TOTAL:				TOTAL:		

Exercise Activity: Hours || Minutes || Calories Burned

Measurements: Weight || Chest || Waist || Hips

How Do I Feel About
My Progress Today?

BREAKFAST			LUNCH		
TIME:			TIME:		
LOCATION:			LOCATION:		
FOOD ITEM	CALORIES	CARBS	FOOD ITEM	CALORIES	CARBS
TOTAL:			TOTAL:		
DINNER			SNACK		
TIME:			TIME:		
LOCATION:			LOCATION:		
FOOD ITEM	CALORIES	CARBS	FOOD ITEM	CALORIES	CARBS
TOTAL:			TOTAL:		

DATE _____

Exercise Activity: Hours || Minutes || Calories Burned

_____

Measurements: Weight || Chest || Waist || Hips

_____

How Do I Feel About
My Progress Today?

BREAKFAST				LUNCH		
TIME:				TIME:		
LOCATION:				LOCATION:		
FOOD ITEM		CALORIES	CARBS	FOOD ITEM		CALORIES	CARBS
TOTAL:				TOTAL:		

DINNER				SNACK		
TIME:				TIME:		
LOCATION:				LOCATION:		
FOOD ITEM		CALORIES	CARBS	FOOD ITEM		CALORIES	CARBS
TOTAL:				TOTAL:		

DATE _____

Exercise Activity: Hours ‖ Minutes ‖ Calories Burned

Measurements: Weight ‖ Chest ‖ Waist ‖ Hips

How Do I Feel About
My Progress Today?

BREAKFAST			LUNCH		
TIME:			TIME:		
LOCATION:			LOCATION:		
FOOD ITEM	CALORIES	CARBS	FOOD ITEM	CALORIES	CARBS
TOTAL:			TOTAL:		
DINNER			**SNACK**		
TIME:			TIME:		
LOCATION:			LOCATION:		
FOOD ITEM	CALORIES	CARBS	FOOD ITEM	CALORIES	CARBS
TOTAL:			TOTAL:		

Exercise Activity: Hours ‖ Minutes ‖ Calories Burned

Measurements: Weight ‖ Chest ‖ Waist ‖ Hips

How Do I Feel About
My Progress Today?

BREAKFAST			LUNCH		
TIME:			TIME:		
LOCATION:			LOCATION:		
FOOD ITEM	CALORIES	CARBS	FOOD ITEM	CALORIES	CARBS
TOTAL:			TOTAL:		

DINNER			SNACK		
TIME:			TIME:		
LOCATION:			LOCATION:		
FOOD ITEM	CALORIES	CARBS	FOOD ITEM	CALORIES	CARBS
TOTAL:			TOTAL:		

Exercise Activity: Hours || Minutes || Calories Burned

Measurements: Weight || Chest || Waist || Hips

How Do I Feel About
My Progress Today?

BREAKFAST			LUNCH		
TIME:			TIME:		
LOCATION:			LOCATION:		
FOOD ITEM	CALORIES	CARBS	FOOD ITEM	CALORIES	CARBS
TOTAL:			TOTAL:		

DINNER			SNACK		
TIME:			TIME:		
LOCATION:			LOCATION:		
FOOD ITEM	CALORIES	CARBS	FOOD ITEM	CALORIES	CARBS
TOTAL:			TOTAL:		

DATE _____

Exercise Activity: Hours || Minutes || Calories Burned

Measurements: Weight || Chest || Waist || Hips

How Do I Feel About
My Progress Today?

BREAKFAST			LUNCH		
TIME:			TIME:		
LOCATION:			LOCATION:		
FOOD ITEM	CALORIES	CARBS	FOOD ITEM	CALORIES	CARBS
TOTAL:			TOTAL:		

DINNER			SNACK		
TIME:			TIME:		
LOCATION:			LOCATION:		
FOOD ITEM	CALORIES	CARBS	FOOD ITEM	CALORIES	CARBS
TOTAL:			TOTAL:		

Exercise Activity: Hours ‖ Minutes ‖ Calories Burned

Measurements: Weight ‖ Chest ‖ Waist ‖ Hips

How Do I Feel About
My Progress Today?

BREAKFAST			LUNCH		
TIME:			TIME:		
LOCATION:			LOCATION:		
FOOD ITEM	CALORIES	CARBS	FOOD ITEM	CALORIES	CARBS
TOTAL:			TOTAL:		

DINNER			SNACK		
TIME:			TIME:		
LOCATION:			LOCATION:		
FOOD ITEM	CALORIES	CARBS	FOOD ITEM	CALORIES	CARBS
TOTAL:			TOTAL:		

DATE _____

Exercise Activity: Hours || Minutes || Calories Burned

Measurements: Weight || Chest || Waist || Hips

How Do I Feel About
My Progress Today?

BREAKFAST			LUNCH		
TIME:			TIME:		
LOCATION:			LOCATION:		
FOOD ITEM	CALORIES	CARBS	FOOD ITEM	CALORIES	CARBS
TOTAL:			TOTAL:		

DINNER			SNACK		
TIME:			TIME:		
LOCATION:			LOCATION:		
FOOD ITEM	CALORIES	CARBS	FOOD ITEM	CALORIES	CARBS
TOTAL:			TOTAL:		

Exercise Activity: Hours || Minutes || Calories Burned

Measurements: Weight || Chest || Waist || Hips

How Do I Feel About
My Progress Today?

BREAKFAST			LUNCH		
TIME:			TIME:		
LOCATION:			LOCATION:		
FOOD ITEM	CALORIES	CARBS	FOOD ITEM	CALORIES	CARBS
TOTAL:			TOTAL:		

DINNER			SNACK		
TIME:			TIME:		
LOCATION:			LOCATION:		
FOOD ITEM	CALORIES	CARBS	FOOD ITEM	CALORIES	CARBS
TOTAL:			TOTAL:		

DATE _____

Exercise Activity: Hours ‖ Minutes ‖ Calories Burned

Measurements: Weight ‖ Chest ‖ Waist ‖ Hips

How Do I Feel About
My Progress Today?

BREAKFAST			LUNCH		
TIME:			TIME:		
LOCATION:			LOCATION:		
FOOD ITEM	CALORIES	CARBS	FOOD ITEM	CALORIES	CARBS
TOTAL:			TOTAL:		

DINNER			SNACK		
TIME:			TIME:		
LOCATION:			LOCATION:		
FOOD ITEM	CALORIES	CARBS	FOOD ITEM	CALORIES	CARBS
TOTAL:			TOTAL:		

Exercise Activity: Hours || Minutes || Calories Burned

Measurements: Weight || Chest || Waist || Hips

How Do I Feel About
My Progress Today?

BREAKFAST			LUNCH		
TIME:			TIME:		
LOCATION:			LOCATION:		
FOOD ITEM	CALORIES	CARBS	FOOD ITEM	CALORIES	CARBS
TOTAL:			TOTAL:		

DINNER			SNACK		
TIME:			TIME:		
LOCATION:			LOCATION:		
FOOD ITEM	CALORIES	CARBS	FOOD ITEM	CALORIES	CARBS
TOTAL:			TOTAL:		

DATE _____

Exercise Activity: Hours || Minutes || Calories Burned

Measurements: Weight || Chest || Waist || Hips

How Do I Feel About My Progress Today?

BREAKFAST			LUNCH		
TIME:			TIME:		
LOCATION:			LOCATION:		
FOOD ITEM	CALORIES	CARBS	FOOD ITEM	CALORIES	CARBS
TOTAL:			TOTAL:		

DINNER			SNACK		
TIME:			TIME:		
LOCATION:			LOCATION:		
FOOD ITEM	CALORIES	CARBS	FOOD ITEM	CALORIES	CARBS
TOTAL:			TOTAL:		

Exercise Activity: Hours || Minutes || Calories Burned

Measurements: Weight || Chest || Waist || Hips

How Do I Feel About
My Progress Today?

BREAKFAST			LUNCH		
TIME:			TIME:		
LOCATION:			LOCATION:		
FOOD ITEM	CALORIES	CARBS	FOOD ITEM	CALORIES	CARBS
TOTAL:			TOTAL:		
DINNER			SNACK		
TIME:			TIME:		
LOCATION:			LOCATION:		
FOOD ITEM	CALORIES	CARBS	FOOD ITEM	CALORIES	CARBS
TOTAL:			TOTAL:		

DATE _____

Exercise Activity: Hours || Minutes || Calories Burned

Measurements: Weight || Chest || Waist || Hips

How Do I Feel About My Progress Today?

BREAKFAST			LUNCH		
TIME:			TIME:		
LOCATION:			LOCATION:		
FOOD ITEM	CALORIES	CARBS	FOOD ITEM	CALORIES	CARBS
TOTAL:			TOTAL:		

DINNER			SNACK		
TIME:			TIME:		
LOCATION:			LOCATION:		
FOOD ITEM	CALORIES	CARBS	FOOD ITEM	CALORIES	CARBS
TOTAL:			TOTAL:		

DATE _____

Exercise Activity: Hours || Minutes || Calories Burned

Measurements: Weight || Chest || Waist || Hips

How Do I Feel About
My Progress Today?

BREAKFAST			LUNCH		
TIME:			TIME:		
LOCATION:			LOCATION:		
FOOD ITEM	CALORIES	CARBS	FOOD ITEM	CALORIES	CARBS
TOTAL:			TOTAL:		

DINNER			SNACK		
TIME:			TIME:		
LOCATION:			LOCATION:		
FOOD ITEM	CALORIES	CARBS	FOOD ITEM	CALORIES	CARBS
TOTAL:			TOTAL:		

DATE _____

Exercise Activity: Hours || Minutes || Calories Burned

Measurements: Weight || Chest || Waist || Hips

How Do I Feel About
My Progress Today?

BREAKFAST			LUNCH		
TIME:			TIME:		
LOCATION:			LOCATION:		
FOOD ITEM	CALORIES	CARBS	FOOD ITEM	CALORIES	CARBS
TOTAL:			TOTAL:		

DINNER			SNACK		
TIME:			TIME:		
LOCATION:			LOCATION:		
FOOD ITEM	CALORIES	CARBS	FOOD ITEM	CALORIES	CARBS
TOTAL:			TOTAL:		

DATE _____

Exercise Activity: Hours || Minutes || Calories Burned

Measurements: Weight || Chest || Waist || Hips

How Do I Feel About
My Progress Today?

BREAKFAST			LUNCH		
TIME:			TIME:		
LOCATION:			LOCATION:		
FOOD ITEM	CALORIES	CARBS	FOOD ITEM	CALORIES	CARBS
TOTAL:			TOTAL:		

DINNER			SNACK		
TIME:			TIME:		
LOCATION:			LOCATION:		
FOOD ITEM	CALORIES	CARBS	FOOD ITEM	CALORIES	CARBS
TOTAL:			TOTAL:		

DATE _____

Exercise Activity: Hours || Minutes || Calories Burned

Measurements: Weight || Chest || Waist || Hips

How Do I Feel About
My Progress Today?

BREAKFAST			LUNCH		
TIME:			TIME:		
LOCATION:			LOCATION:		
FOOD ITEM	CALORIES	CARBS	FOOD ITEM	CALORIES	CARBS
TOTAL:			TOTAL:		
DINNER			**SNACK**		
TIME:			TIME:		
LOCATION:			LOCATION:		
FOOD ITEM	CALORIES	CARBS	FOOD ITEM	CALORIES	CARBS
TOTAL:			TOTAL:		

Exercise Activity: Hours || Minutes || Calories Burned

Measurements: Weight || Chest || Waist || Hips

How Do I Feel About
My Progress Today?

BREAKFAST			LUNCH		
TIME:			TIME:		
LOCATION:			LOCATION:		
FOOD ITEM	CALORIES	CARBS	FOOD ITEM	CALORIES	CARBS
TOTAL:			TOTAL:		

DINNER			SNACK		
TIME:			TIME:		
LOCATION:			LOCATION:		
FOOD ITEM	CALORIES	CARBS	FOOD ITEM	CALORIES	CARBS
TOTAL:			TOTAL:		

Exercise Activity: Hours || Minutes || Calories Burned

Measurements: Weight || Chest || Waist || Hips

How Do I Feel About
My Progress Today?

BREAKFAST			LUNCH		
TIME:			TIME:		
LOCATION:			LOCATION:		
FOOD ITEM	CALORIES	CARBS	FOOD ITEM	CALORIES	CARBS
TOTAL:			TOTAL:		

DINNER			SNACK		
TIME:			TIME:		
LOCATION:			LOCATION:		
FOOD ITEM	CALORIES	CARBS	FOOD ITEM	CALORIES	CARBS
TOTAL:			TOTAL:		

Exercise Activity: Hours || Minutes || Calories Burned

Measurements: Weight || Chest || Waist || Hips

How Do I Feel About
My Progress Today?

BREAKFAST			LUNCH		
TIME:			TIME:		
LOCATION:			LOCATION:		
FOOD ITEM	CALORIES	CARBS	FOOD ITEM	CALORIES	CARBS
TOTAL:			TOTAL:		

DINNER			SNACK		
TIME:			TIME:		
LOCATION:			LOCATION:		
FOOD ITEM	CALORIES	CARBS	FOOD ITEM	CALORIES	CARBS
TOTAL:			TOTAL:		

DATE _____

Exercise Activity: Hours ‖ Minutes ‖ Calories Burned

Measurements: Weight ‖ Chest ‖ Waist ‖ Hips

How Do I Feel About My Progress Today?

BREAKFAST			LUNCH		
TIME:			TIME:		
LOCATION:			LOCATION:		
FOOD ITEM	CALORIES	CARBS	FOOD ITEM	CALORIES	CARBS
TOTAL:			TOTAL:		

DINNER			SNACK		
TIME:			TIME:		
LOCATION:			LOCATION:		
FOOD ITEM	CALORIES	CARBS	FOOD ITEM	CALORIES	CARBS
TOTAL:			TOTAL:		

Exercise Activity: Hours || Minutes || Calories Burned

Measurements: Weight || Chest || Waist || Hips

How Do I Feel About
My Progress Today?

BREAKFAST			LUNCH		
TIME:			TIME:		
LOCATION:			LOCATION:		
FOOD ITEM	CALORIES	CARBS	FOOD ITEM	CALORIES	CARBS
TOTAL:			TOTAL:		

DINNER			SNACK		
TIME:			TIME:		
LOCATION:			LOCATION:		
FOOD ITEM	CALORIES	CARBS	FOOD ITEM	CALORIES	CARBS
TOTAL:			TOTAL:		

Exercise Activity: Hours ‖ Minutes ‖ Calories Burned

Measurements: Weight ‖ Chest ‖ Waist ‖ Hips

How Do I Feel About
My Progress Today?

BREAKFAST			**LUNCH**		
TIME:			TIME:		
LOCATION:			LOCATION:		
FOOD ITEM	CALORIES	CARBS	FOOD ITEM	CALORIES	CARBS
TOTAL:			TOTAL:		
DINNER			**SNACK**		
TIME:			TIME:		
LOCATION:			LOCATION:		
FOOD ITEM	CALORIES	CARBS	FOOD ITEM	CALORIES	CARBS
TOTAL:			TOTAL:		

DATE _____

Exercise Activity: Hours || Minutes || Calories Burned

Measurements: Weight || Chest || Waist || Hips

How Do I Feel About
My Progress Today?

BREAKFAST			LUNCH		
TIME:			TIME:		
LOCATION:			LOCATION:		
FOOD ITEM	CALORIES	CARBS	FOOD ITEM	CALORIES	CARBS
TOTAL:			TOTAL:		

DINNER			SNACK		
TIME:			TIME:		
LOCATION:			LOCATION:		
FOOD ITEM	CALORIES	CARBS	FOOD ITEM	CALORIES	CARBS
TOTAL:			TOTAL:		

Exercise Activity: Hours || Minutes || Calories Burned

Measurements: Weight || Chest || Waist || Hips

How Do I Feel About
My Progress Today?

BREAKFAST			**LUNCH**		
TIME:			TIME:		
LOCATION:			LOCATION:		
FOOD ITEM	CALORIES	CARBS	FOOD ITEM	CALORIES	CARBS
TOTAL:			TOTAL:		
DINNER			**SNACK**		
TIME:			TIME:		
LOCATION:			LOCATION:		
FOOD ITEM	CALORIES	CARBS	FOOD ITEM	CALORIES	CARBS
TOTAL:			TOTAL:		

DATE _____

Exercise Activity: Hours || Minutes || Calories Burned

Measurements: Weight || Chest || Waist || Hips

How Do I Feel About
My Progress Today?

BREAKFAST			LUNCH		
TIME:			TIME:		
LOCATION:			LOCATION:		
FOOD ITEM	CALORIES	CARBS	FOOD ITEM	CALORIES	CARBS
TOTAL:			TOTAL:		

DINNER			SNACK		
TIME:			TIME:		
LOCATION:			LOCATION:		
FOOD ITEM	CALORIES	CARBS	FOOD ITEM	CALORIES	CARBS
TOTAL:			TOTAL:		

DATE _____

Exercise Activity: Hours || Minutes || Calories Burned

_____

Measurements: Weight || Chest || Waist || Hips

_____

How Do I Feel About
My Progress Today?

BREAKFAST			LUNCH		
TIME:			TIME:		
LOCATION:			LOCATION:		
FOOD ITEM	CALORIES	CARBS	FOOD ITEM	CALORIES	CARBS
TOTAL:			TOTAL:		

DINNER			SNACK		
TIME:			TIME:		
LOCATION:			LOCATION:		
FOOD ITEM	CALORIES	CARBS	FOOD ITEM	CALORIES	CARBS
TOTAL:			TOTAL:		

Exercise Activity: Hours || Minutes || Calories Burned

Measurements: Weight || Chest || Waist || Hips

How Do I Feel About My Progress Today?

BREAKFAST			LUNCH		
TIME:			TIME:		
LOCATION:			LOCATION:		
FOOD ITEM	CALORIES	CARBS	FOOD ITEM	CALORIES	CARBS
TOTAL:			TOTAL:		

DINNER			SNACK		
TIME:			TIME:		
LOCATION:			LOCATION:		
FOOD ITEM	CALORIES	CARBS	FOOD ITEM	CALORIES	CARBS
TOTAL:			TOTAL:		

DATE _____

Exercise Activity: Hours || Minutes || Calories Burned

Measurements: Weight || Chest || Waist || Hips

How Do I Feel About
My Progress Today?

BREAKFAST			LUNCH		
TIME:			TIME:		
LOCATION:			LOCATION:		
FOOD ITEM	CALORIES	CARBS	FOOD ITEM	CALORIES	CARBS
TOTAL:			TOTAL:		

DINNER			SNACK		
TIME:			TIME:		
LOCATION:			LOCATION:		
FOOD ITEM	CALORIES	CARBS	FOOD ITEM	CALORIES	CARBS
TOTAL:			TOTAL:		

DATE _____

Exercise Activity: Hours || Minutes || Calories Burned

Measurements: Weight || Chest || Waist || Hips

How Do I Feel About
My Progress Today?

BREAKFAST			LUNCH		
TIME:			TIME:		
LOCATION:			LOCATION:		
FOOD ITEM	CALORIES	CARBS	FOOD ITEM	CALORIES	CARBS
TOTAL:			TOTAL:		

DINNER			SNACK		
TIME:			TIME:		
LOCATION:			LOCATION:		
FOOD ITEM	CALORIES	CARBS	FOOD ITEM	CALORIES	CARBS
TOTAL:			TOTAL:		

NOTES:

NOTES:

NOTES:

NOTES:

Made in the USA
Coppell, TX
10 January 2023